BEHAVIOURAL DISORDERS
IN DOGS AND CATS

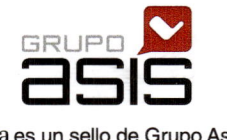

Dedicated to all the animals that have accompanied me through life's journey and helped me appreciate the strength of the emotional bond that humans can establish with them.

With a special dedication to my first animal, Negra, a mixed-breed stray whom I found so long ago that I cannot even remember where; she was responsible for awakening my interest and affection for animals. And to Atenea, my current dog, whom I also found in the street; she represents all the animals I have shared my life with and which have sparked, and continue fuelling, my desire to learn more about animal behaviour.

Dedicated to the people who have accompanied and supported me, and who are still doing so, while walking this path of discovery.

ACKNOWLEDGEMENTS

It is always hard to write the acknowledgements upon completing a book. There is usually a lot of people, institutions, and companies who you wish to thank for their support, and you are always afraid of leaving someone out.

Fortunately, on this occasion, it has been relatively straightforward with respect to institutions and companies, as I would just like to thank Grupo Asís Biomedia for placing their trust in me to elaborate this guide to normal behaviour and behavioural disorders in dogs and cats.

However, when it comes to people, this is not so easy because there are so many people I must thank for their support. First of all, I would like to express my gratitude to all the veterinary surgeons who, over many years, have referred their patients with behavioural problems to me; secondly, to my nearest and dearest, to whom I was unable to dedicate as much time as they deserve while writing this guide; and lastly, to my patients who, although unaware of their contribution, gave me the chance to accumulate enough experience to bring together in this book.

Finally, I would also like to thank all of you who are taking the time to read this guide.

My sincere thanks to each and every one of you,

Ricardo Luis Bruno Cazeaux

AGRADECIMIENTOS

AUTHOR

RICARDO LUIS BRUNO CAZEAUX

Ricardo Luis Bruno completed his degree in veterinary medicine at the Faculty of Veterinary Sciences, University of Buenos Aires (Argentina), and is licenced in veterinary practice (Spain) by the Office of Degrees and Recognition of Qualifications at the Spanish Ministry of Education's General Directorate for University Policy. He was awarded the title of Specialist in Animal Behaviour by the Argentinian Professional Board of Veterinarians and earned a master's in Animal Behaviour and Ecology from the Universidad de los Pueblos de Europa (Spain).

He has previously worked as a veterinary surgeon in animal behaviour for Pro Animale, a German animal protection society, and in 2003, 2004, and 2009, Ricardo was in charge of a dog shelter in Ayvalik (Turkey) subsidised by Pro Animale with a population of 1,200 dogs.

Ricardo has acted as a technical consultant and development manager for the first medicine manufactured in Argentina for the treatment of behavioural disorders in pets.

He has been a guest lecturer at the Tandil Faculty of Veterinary Sciences, attached to the National University of Central Buenos Aires, and was responsible for the Animal Behaviour module as part of the academic intensification course, under the supervision of the Small Animal Veterinary Surgery Department.

Ricardo has served as a full member of the assessment panel for the title of specialist in clinical veterinary medicine in cats and dogs awarded by the Santa Fe Provincial College of Veterinary Surgeons (Argentina).

He designed the study programme and was co-coordinator and lecturer for a specialist course on domestic cat and dog behaviour organised by the Faculty of Veterinary at the Universidad Nacional de La Plata (Argentina).

He also developed the study programme and lectured as part of the International Online (e-learning) Course in Companion Animal Behaviour – a 13-week long course organised by the veterinary portal Vet Praxis in Peru. Ricardo has also lectured as part of the International Online Diploma Course in Clinical Animal Behaviour organised by VEPA (Association of Small Animal Veterinarians) in the department of Antioquia, Colombia.

Since 2013, he has been a lecturer of the Cat Behaviour module for the international online postgraduate course on feline medicine, imparted through the veterinary IT portal *www.veterinariosenweb.com* belonging to the Universidad Católica de Salta (Argentina).

He is a coauthor of *Medicina felina práctica II* (Practical Feline Medicine II) and collaborated on *Consulta rápida en la clínica diaria* (Rapid Consultations in Everyday Clinical Practice). Ricardo Luis elaborated the study material on animal welfare, zoonoses, and canine and feline behaviour for the 2007 TACA course (animal-assisted therapy) imparted at the Faculty of Veterinary Sciences, University of Buenos Aires (Argentina).

He wrote the book *Una guía para entender a tu gato* (A Guide to Understanding your Cat) (Editorial Grijalbo, Penguin Random House Grupo Editorial, 2017) aimed at the general public.

Since 2018, he has created content for the digital communication strategy of a company in the sector.

Author's website *www.conductismoanimal.com.ar.*

PREFACE

Within the field of small animal medicine, animal behaviour is a relatively new field that still needs to be explored a lot more, but it is also one with a bright future ahead. The current interest of society in animal behaviour has led to animal owners being increasingly interested in knowing what behaviour patterns are normal in their animals. In addition, as the urban population increases, so does the number of animals that cannot perform all their innate behaviour patterns and therefore engage in inappropriate behaviours due to frustration.

In this specialty, it is important to work with responsible owners, who have time and are willing to play an active role in the therapy to improve their animal's behavioural disorder. Knowledge in this field is still limited among the general population and, what is worse, people have access to a lot of incomplete or incorrect information about animal behaviour. Solving this issue is mostly the responsibility of veterinary professionals and leaving this task in the hands of other professionals should, at least in my opinion, almost be considered malpractice.

Companion animal behaviour often remains a forgotten aspect of veterinary medicine. Usually, the owners of a puppy or kitten are given recommendations about vaccines and their animal's general care, diet and hygiene, but they receive little advice on the typical behaviours in their pet's species and what they can do to ensure they enjoy life together. Sometimes animal behaviour is even left in the hands of people who are not animal health professionals and who may not be qualified to provide advice on this topic.

This book aims at helping small animal (cats and dogs) vets develop a greater understanding of animal behaviour. It is scientifically rigorous and provides an experience-based approach to dealing with real-life cases.

Ricardo Luis Bruno Cazeaux

TABLE OF CONTENTS

BEHAVIOURAL DISORDERS IN DOGS

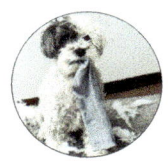

DISORDERS ASSOCIATED WITH ANXIETY AND STRESS

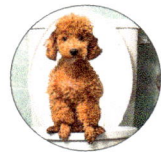

DISORDERS ASSOCIATED WITH ELIMINATION BEHAVIOUR

BEHAVIOURAL DISORDERS IN CATS

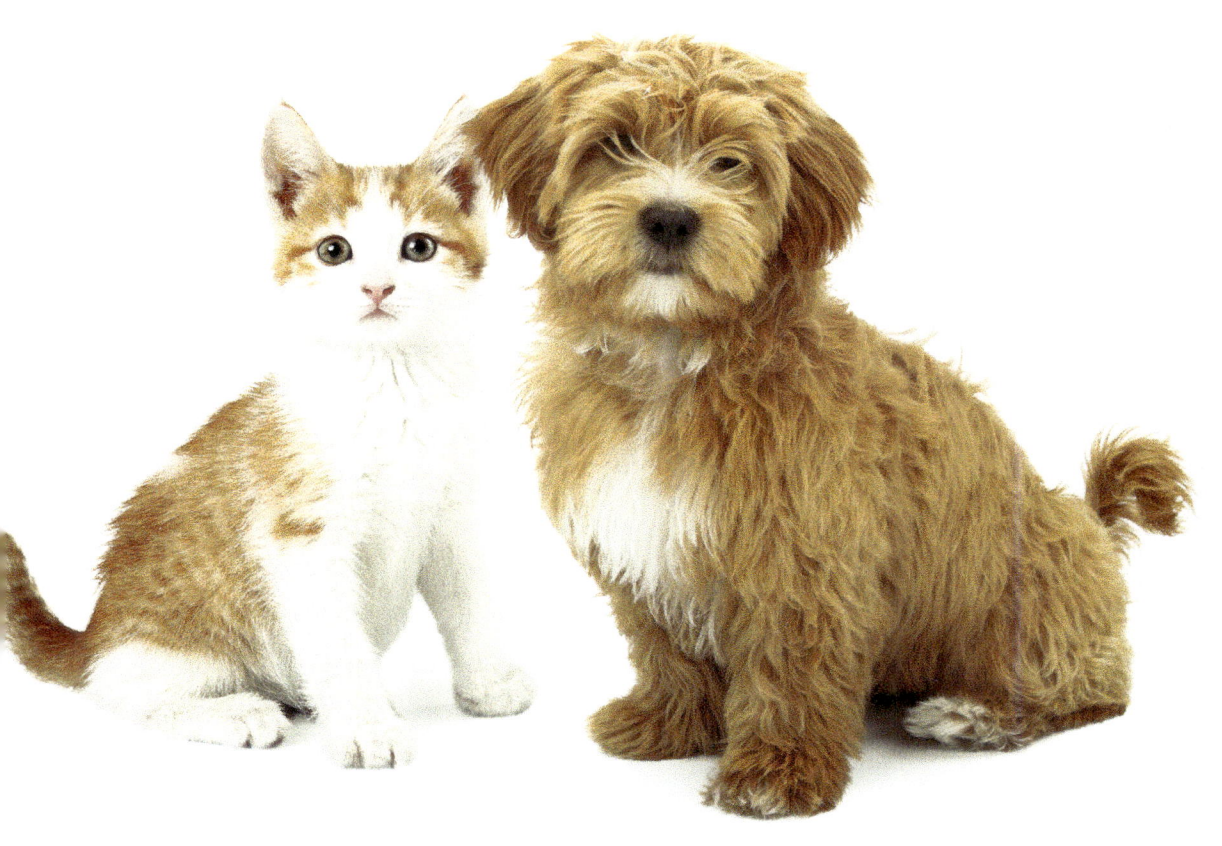

BEHAVIOURAL DISORDERS
IN DOGS

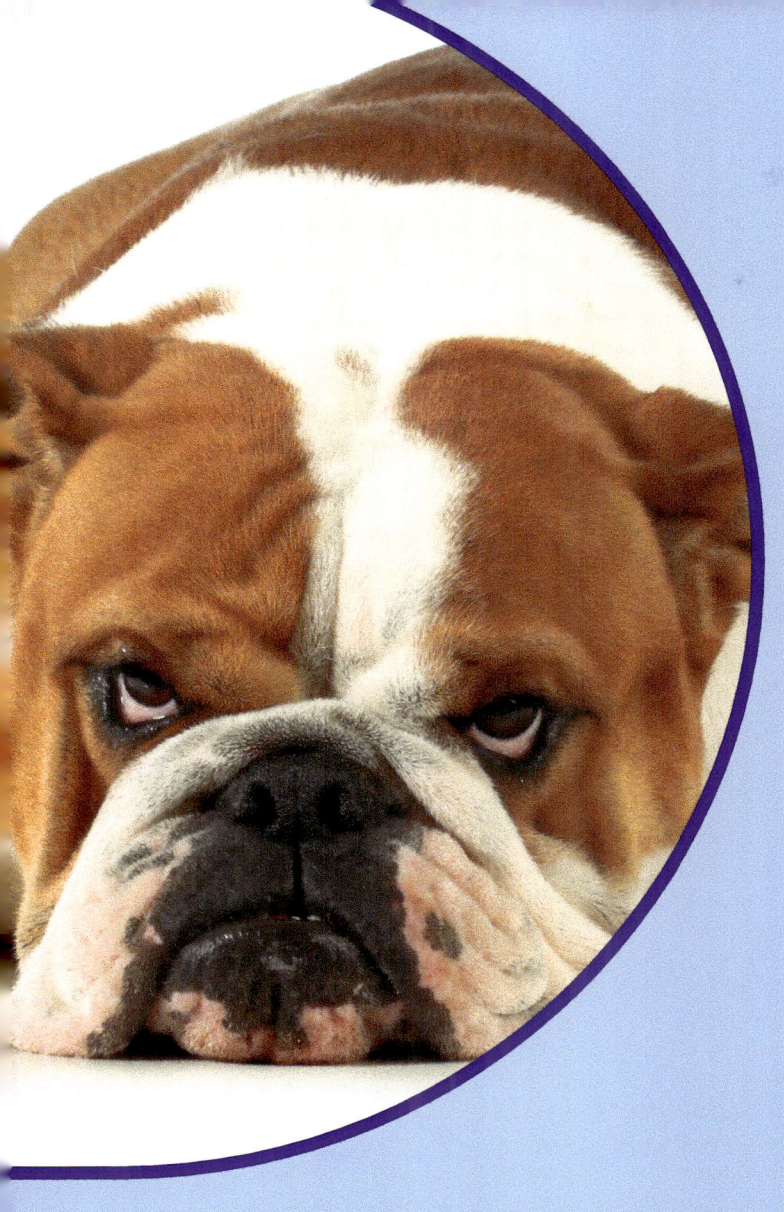

READ ME FIRST

BEHAVIOURAL DISORDERS IN DOGS

An animal's behaviour is the product of the interaction of many different variables: genetic factors, early life experiences, learnings, physiological condition, and environmental stimuli.

> All behaviours have both a genetic and an environmental component.

Members of each species follow their own specific behavioural patterns which they develop and adapt to their natural habitat based on early experiences and learnings. Veterinary surgeons must be familiar with these patterns so they can differentiate them from abnormal or nonadaptive behaviours. To understand normal canine behaviour, we first need to have a look at its ancestor – the Asian Grey Wolf – with whom dogs share 99.8 % of their mitochondrial DNA and basic behavioural patterns.

Wolves are gregarious animals that form packs with a strict and intricate pyramidal social organisation in which an alpha wolf rules over various beta, gamma, and delta individuals (Fig. 1). This dominant–subordinate relationship can change depending on the circumstances. Similarly, animals beneath the leader can dominate or be dominated by others in the pack.

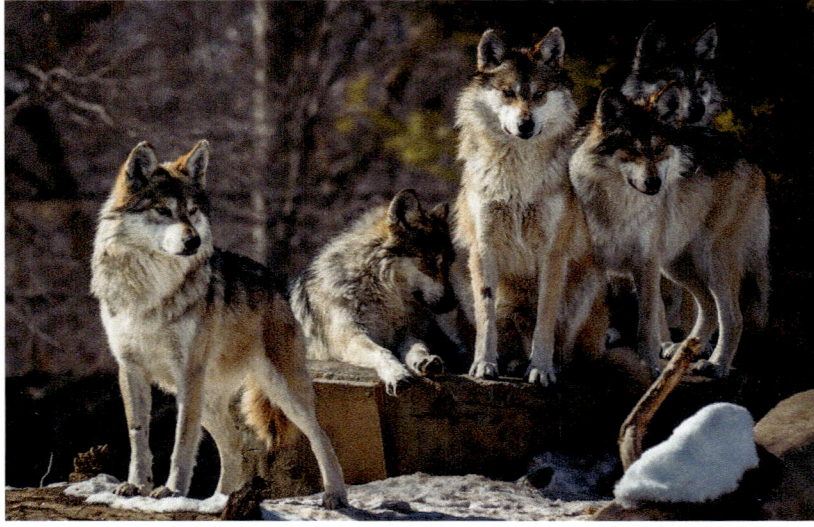

Figure 1. Wolves, the direct ancestors of dogs, are a very sociable species.

Wolves are highly adapted to exercise and can cover up to 45 km a day in search of prey. They have also developed an effective, complicated, and varied communication system built around specific gestures, attitudes, postures, and behaviours. The most important of these are threatening and aggressive postures and attitudes, which are often displayed when a subordinate animal challenges a superior and, if it emerges victorious, takes up a new position in the pack's hierarchy. This point is very important because it forms the foundation for one of the most commonly encountered behavioural alterations in domestic pet dogs: dominance aggression.

Dogs and wolves share some common characteristics:

➤ They are highly sociable and make use of an excellent and sophisticated communication system to interact with the rest of their pack.
➤ They have adapted to spend 80 % of their time in close contact with their social group.
➤ They follow a hierarchy that is strictly respected, but which is open to change through force and aggression.
➤ They both have an athletic body adapted to trekking long distances (Fig. 2).

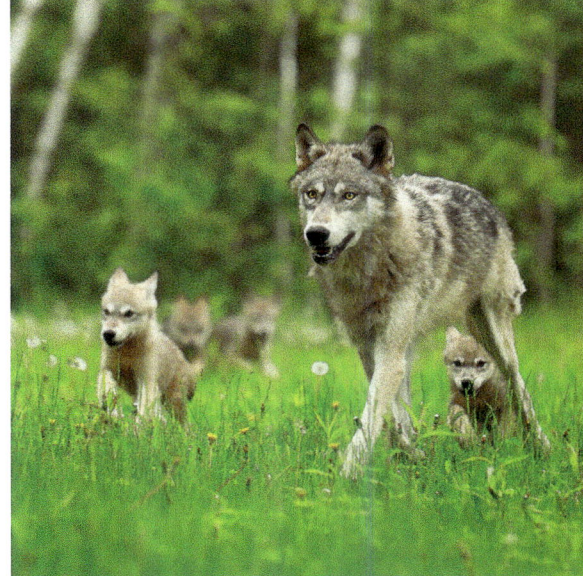

Figure 2. Wolves and dogs both have athletic bodies that are well-adapted to covering long distances.

These concepts must be taken into account when trying to understand behavioural problems in pet dogs, as a high percentage of such alterations are rooted in dogs being prohibited from expressing the inherited behavioural patterns that are normal for their species.

A healthy and well-balanced dog can develop, execute, and exhibit typical behavioural patterns expected of its species.

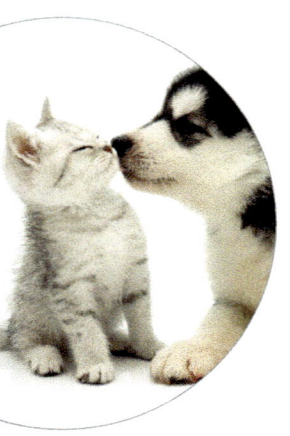

BEHAVIOURAL DEVELOPMENT

Puppyhood represents an essential stage that will influence the dog's future life, since most behavioural disorders that might later arise in adult dogs take root during this period. Puppies go through four well-defined stages of behavioural development:

➤ **Neonatal:** this phase spans a dog's first 2 weeks of life. Due to the neurophysiological immaturity of newborn puppies, their behaviour is limited to infantile patterns consisting mainly of sleeping and nursing. Puppies are born with their eyes and ear canals closed, so they are totally dependent on their mothers. Defaecation and urination are involuntary reflex actions that are only provoked by tactile stimulation of a puppy's anogenital area.

➤ **Transitional:** this stage covers puppies aged from 14 to 21 days. At this point, puppies start to explore their surroundings and practise using their motor skills. The advancing development of their limbs, sight, and hearing gives pups the opportunity to investigate their immediate environment, initially crawling along the floor before walking in an uncoordinated manner. In the third week of life puppies start accumulating experiences that will condition their future behaviour. By this age, researchers have observed slow-wave sleep patterns in electroencephalograms (EEG). Elimination behaviour is no longer exclusively a reflex action.

IMPRINTING PERIOD

Imprinting is the process by which an animal learns to recognise its parents' characteristics and, by extension, the characteristics of other members of its species, particularly the constituents of its own social group. Imprinting occurs at an undefined time between the first and second stages.

➤ **Socialisation:** this period begins when puppies have minimally functional senses and well-developed motor function, and while it spans from 3 weeks to 12–15 weeks, the young dog's experiences in weeks 5 to 8 are particularly crucial. This stage sees the appearance of several different traits in terms of the animal's physical, neurological, and behavioural maturation. The nervous system starts to mature and puppies commence a phase of stable learning and motor development, which means they begin to display specific behaviours and form their personality. They also start to interact with each other, at first playfully, but this quickly turns into fighting, ambushes, growling, and tug-of-war over objects. Studies indicate the importance of this period in creating attachment to people, places, and eating habits. It is the most important stage of puppyhood, when individuals learn to recognise other animals (Fig. 3). Similarly, a wide range of behavioural alterations, which can be very hard to correct in adulthood, begin to develop in this stage. Negative experiences at this age can result in inappropriate socialisation.

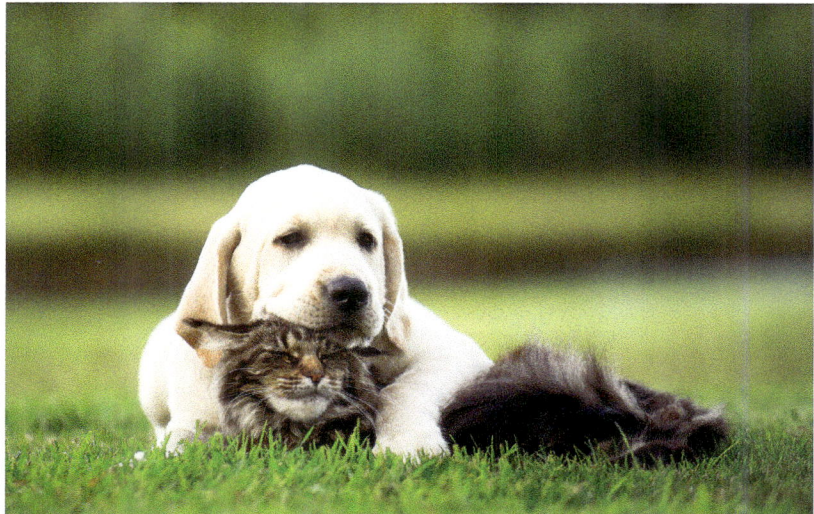

Figure 3. Puppies learn to recognise other animals during the socialisation stage of their development.

➤ **Adolescence:** this stage extends from the end of the socialisation period until the animal has fully developed and reached maturity, depending on individual variations such as sex, breed, and so on. By this age, puppies have already created social bonds and learnt typical canine behavioural patterns, so they now spend a lot of time exploring their surroundings (Fig. 4). Adolescent dogs occasionally need to revisit everything they have learnt in the socialisation period to help commit it to memory. Their basic learning capacity is fully developed, but the rate at which they assimilate new skills starts to decline because they rely more heavily on previous learnings. While it is true, from a behavioural perspective, that this stage is not as important as the socialisation phase, it is still very significant because many aggressive behavioural disorders observed in adult dogs tend to initially appear during adolescence. From the age of 8–12 months when dogs approach sexual maturity, particularly males under the influence of testicular hormone secretions, they generally start to display more aggressiveness and try to position themselves in their social hierarchy using threats and aggressive attitudes.

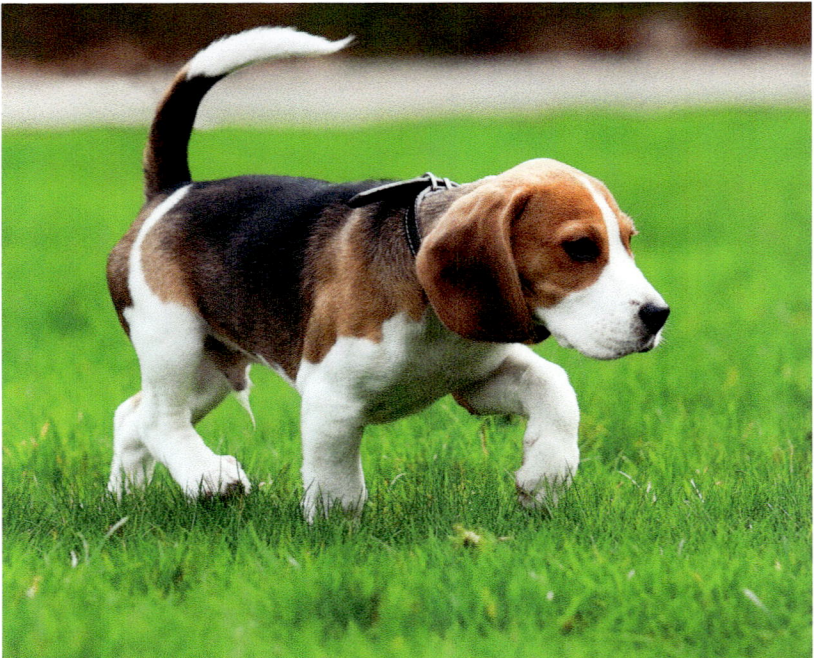

Figure 4. During adolescence, puppies actively explore their surroundings.

> Dogs reach behavioural maturity at twice the age of sexual maturity (first oestrus in females and ability to ejaculate in the case of males).

THE IMPORTANCE OF SOCIALISATION

During the socialisation period, puppies get used to the environment in which they will presumably spend the rest of their lives and learn to develop in it without fear, mistrust, or insecurity. They also learn how to interact with other dogs and individuals from other species (Box 1). Ultimately, socialisation is when dogs achieve optimal adaptation to the habitat and conditions in which they will live.

This period is particularly important because it is when many different potential behavioural disorders start to germinate and these will be hard to correct when the dog is an adult.

It is essential for puppies to have contact with other dogs during this period (Fig. 5), otherwise they cannot continue to learn appropriate canine behavioural patterns, plus they might develop phobias or aggressive conducts in the future.

The socialisation stage is when puppies start to develop their ability to quickly associate behaviours with specific stimuli, so it is also when their education should begin with specific lessons (teaching them to eliminate outside, obey simple orders, etc.). Similarly, puppies easily fix on any negative occurrences they might experience, which could mean that animals find it hard to adapt to their environment in subsequent stages of their lives.

Puppies should not be subject to excessively long periods of social isolation, as they run the risk of losing the progress gained from previous social experiences which is necessary for optimal behavioural development.

Box 1. Socialisation stage of puppyhood.

Age in weeks					
1–2	3–5	6–9	10–11	12–14	15
▲ Puppies should remain with their mother and littermates. ▲ Expose them to the smell of humans, both men and women. ▲ They should be handled gently and with particular care.	▲ Puppies should receive interesting and nonthreatening stimuli. ▲ Expose them to household noises such as the washing machine, vacuum cleaner, and so on. ▲ Start to habituate puppies to the normal household environment. ▲ They should continue to interact with their littermates.	▲ This is when puppies usually start their lives with their new owner(s). ▲ They should meet everyone in the family (adults, children, other animals, etc.). ▲ Introduce them to simple situations and activities: brushing their coat, simulated veterinary check-ups, travelling in the car, amongst others. ▲ Accustom them to different types of visitors such as family friends, the postman, and other animals. ▲ Start ignoring them from time to time. ▲ Add food to its bowl while the puppy is eating.	▲ Introduce stronger stimuli (loud noises, agglomerations, etc.). ▲ Start training with a collar. ▲ Initiate socialisation classes with veterinary supervision. ▲ Begin exposure to controlled risks. ▲ Continue to apply the recommendations from the previous stage.	▲ Increase the variety of experiences. ▲ Do not forget that all the training performed until now serves as a means of communication and establishing a relationship with the puppy, they are not one-off guidelines that the dog will learn and apply automatically. ▲ Remember that each dog is a unique individual and they do not necessarily conform to a standard just because they belong to a certain breed.	▲ The puppy has completed the critical socialisation period. ▲ Although the sensitisation period lasts until the age of 12–15 weeks, it is important to reinforce everything learnt to date, otherwise the animal may forget it. Reinforcement training should continue until the dog reaches social maturity after approximately 12 months.

> Some vaccinations on the market provide correct immunisation before puppies reach the end of the socialisation stage.

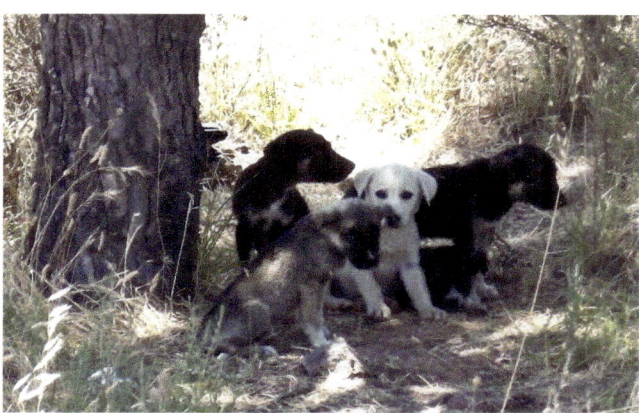

Figure 5. It is essential for puppies to have contact with other dogs during the socialisation stage of puppyhood.

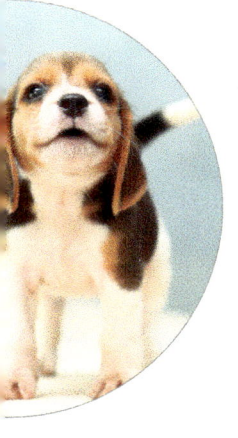

BASIC PUPPY HANDLING AND TRAINING

A lot of future behavioural problems can be avoided in adult dogs if owners follow some simple recommendations during puppyhood. However, the veterinary surgeon is responsible for passing this information to owners.

BEFORE TAKING A PUPPY HOME FOR THE FIRST TIME

Before future owners decide to take on the responsibility of owning a dog, vets should inform them that they need to:

➤ Seriously assess whether they are in a position to own a dog (time, money, patience, etc.).

➤ Remember that mixed-breed dogs generally suffer fewer behavioural problems than pure breeds.

- Get advice about which type of dog (breed, sex, age, etc.) would be most suitable based on the characteristics of their home, family dynamics, and lifestyle.
- Avoid getting a puppy if their previous dog died recently. If they do, the new dog should, where possible, be a different breed, sex, or colour and not have a strong physical resemblance to the old dog.
- Consider, if they already own a dog, that adults can be aggressive towards each other, especially if they are the same sex.
- Remember that aggression is a very common behavioural problem seen in dogs, affecting a high proportion of males.
- Take into account that the ideal age for introducing a puppy to a new home is 6–8 weeks.

PUPPIES AGED 45 DAYS TO 6 MONTHS

Here are some guidelines for handling puppies aged 45 days to 6 months:
- Never punish or scold puppies excessively or for prolonged periods. Any reprimands must be immediate, brief, occasional, and strictly verbal.
- Right from day one, place the puppy in its bed in the owner's bedroom, then after a few days start conditioning it to sleep in its designated place in the home. Puppies are often used to sleeping close to their mothers and littermates, so it is a good idea to place a dog-sized stuffed toy in its bed for the first few days.
- From the outset, puppies should be brought into contact with the different people and animals (other dogs, cats, etc.) they will later encounter in adulthood.
- Calling the puppy by its name when playing will help it learn to recognise it. Do not accustom puppies to an idle lifestyle. Do not take part in competitive games (wrestling, tug-of-war with rags, etc.).
- Do not cuddle or caress puppies excessively. Nor should owners constantly carry them in their arms.
- Walks should be taken 15–30 minutes after puppies have eaten. Since this is when they usually urinate and defaecate, there is a greater chance the animal will eliminate any waste during its walk.

➤ While puppies are still very young and cannot be taken for a walk, owners should designate an area for eliminations away from other areas of activity such as where they play, eat, and so on. Once chosen, owners should avoid changing the location.
➤ Do not allocate the responsibility of caring for the puppy to children or adolescents.
➤ Owners should be made to appreciate that dogs do not have human feelings (hate, resentment, retaliation, love, etc.), rather they have different behavioural patterns.
➤ Get the animal used to wearing a collar and learn to use them correctly.
➤ Do not allow children in the house to constantly irritate and bother puppies.

BASIC TRAINING

The minimum training a puppy should receive from its owner, regardless of whether they decide to turn to a professional trainer, consists of basic obedience exercises.

Training or teaching a dog some basic commands is not just a question of technique, but above all the right attitude. Training should be accompanied by correct routine interaction with the dog.

Owners should avoid giving puppies food to reinforce compliance with orders, as this introduces the risk of triggering a compulsive behaviour with respect to food.

> Two fundamental expressions puppies must understand: "no" and "good dog".

FIRST WALKS WITH A NEW PUPPY

A puppy's first few walks should be used to build up the animal's confidence in the environment, allowing it to smell things and relax. If the puppy is scared by cars, other dogs, and so on, owners should ignore this behaviour, in so far as possible, and continue walking as if everything is normal. Never return home while the dog is still scared by something that happened in the street.

THE "NO" COMMAND

The purpose of this order is to suppress the exhibition of a specific behaviour. Once the animal has learnt the order, it is down to the owner to use it in the appropriate situations. If the puppy does something it should not, the owner should say "no" vigorously but not aggressively.

THE "SIT" COMMAND

This is a straightforward but very useful exercise, as the sitting position can be used in various circumstances: before receiving a reward, to calm a dog over-excited by the presence of a person or another animal, when you want it to wait for a few minutes, and so on.

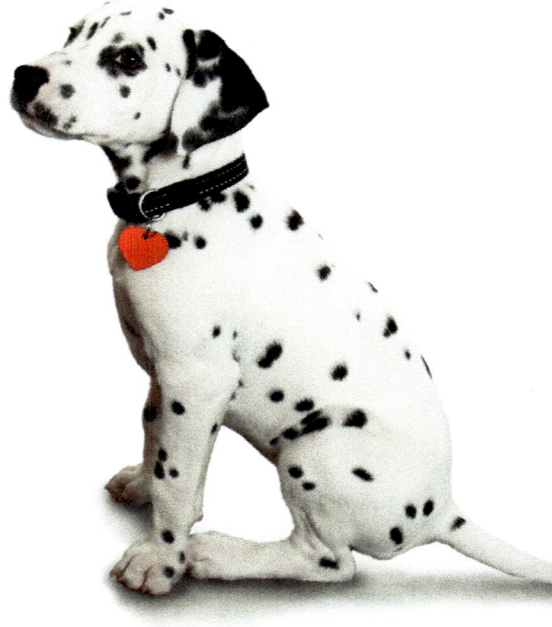

To teach a puppy to sit, take the lead in your right hand and pull upwards while pushing your left hand down gently but firmly on the dog's rump and clearly repeating the order "sit". Congratulate the puppy enthusiastically the first time it executes the command correctly.

WALKING TO HEEL

This is one of the most important skills to teach, and not just because it helps establish the owner's dominance over the animal. It is also indispensable to ensure owners do not lose the will to take their dog out because it pulls too much, which would result in a sedentary lifestyle and undoubtedly future behavioural problems.

Start walking with the puppy and when it begins to pull in front, the owner should issue a few short, gentle tugs on the lead while repeating the command "heel".

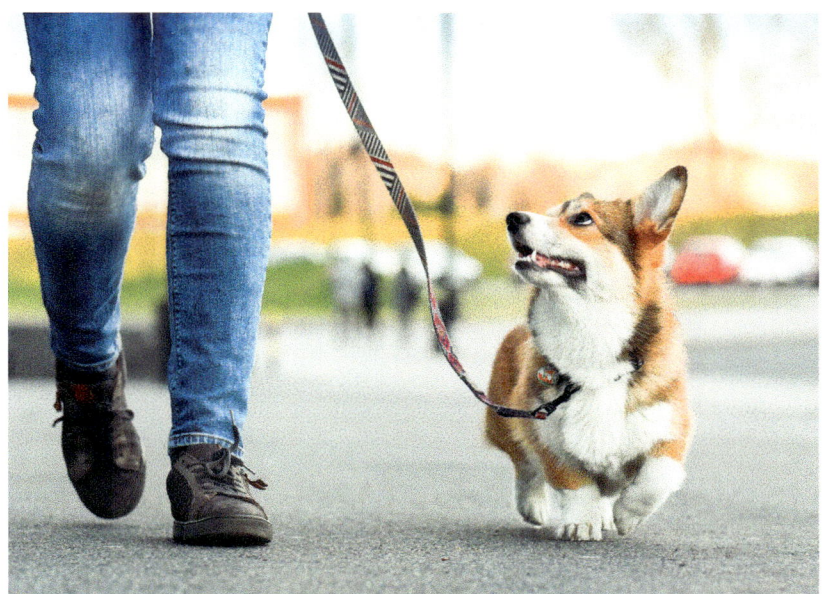

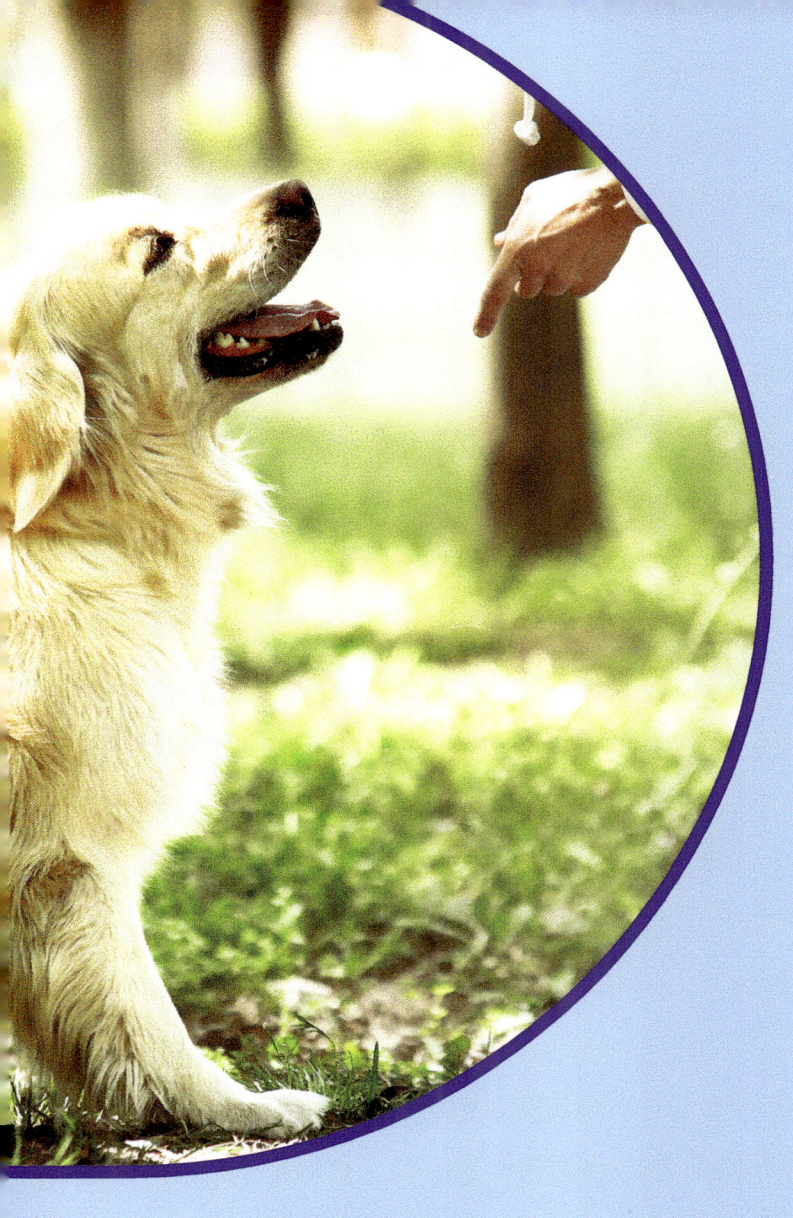

DISORDERS ASSOCIATED WITH AGGRESSIVE BEHAVIOUR

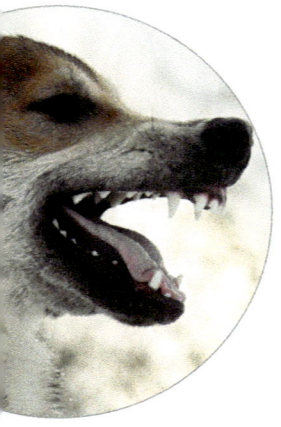

INTRODUCTION

Aggression-related problems are the most common cause for consultation with respect to behavioural alterations in dogs and the second leading cause in cats, which underlines their importance.

As with other behavioural disorders, a patient can be deemed to have an aggression-related behavioural problem when the dog's conduct affects its own or its cohabitants' quality of life.

It is very important to make a precise diagnosis of the type of aggression displayed by the animal. There are various types of aggressive behaviour and, accordingly, each has a different treatment and prognosis.

Aggression is a valuable survival tool for any animal, whether exhibited towards members of the same species or other species (Fig. 1). As such, aggression in itself should not be considered a behavioural disorder, as it corresponds to normal behaviour; nevertheless, it can impact on the dog's peaceful coexistence with other members of the household or it may deviate from typical conduct.

> Aggression, which is exhibited within the same species, should not be misconstrued for predation, which is exercised between different species. The former involves competition that is absent from the latter.

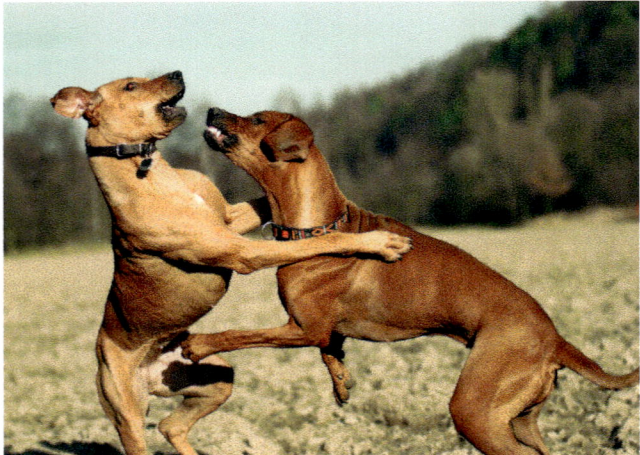

Figure 1. Aggressive behaviour is a survival tool, even between members of the same species.

PATHOPHYSIOLOGY

Some researchers in the fields of neuroscience and experimental neurology currently align with the concept that different regions of the brain correspond to the anatomical and physiological foundations that give rise to aggressive behaviour.

AGGRESSIVE BEHAVIOUR IS REGULATED BY THE LIMBIC SYSTEM

The area of the brain that is generally associated with acts of aggression is called the limbic system. This region of the brain, also known as the visceral or reptilian brain or archicerebellum, is considered a primitive structure in comparison with the dense layer of cells called grey matter, neocortex, or neocerebellum.

The limbic system forms a ring around the inner surface of the brain, the anterior inferior portion of which is known as the amygdala. The amygdala is located deep inside each temporal lobe and has been closely linked to aggressive behaviour.

The cerebral cortex acts on the hypothalamus and amygdala, then these structures affect the midbrain, which finally triggers the animal's display of aggression.

We know that when certain areas of the brain are stimulated it evokes a violent or aggressive response regardless of the situation, context, or subject's previous experience, so these areas constitute the underlying neuronal cause of aggression.

Laboratory studies have shown that electrical stimulation of the dorsal hypothalamic area elicits defensive behaviour, stimulation of the medial hypothalamus induces offensive behaviour, and, lastly, a controlled electrical discharge on the lateral hypothalamus triggers a predatory conduct in test animals.

NEUROTRANSMITTERS

The main neurotransmitter involved in aggressive behaviour is serotonin. Studies have demonstrated that a decrease in a subject's serotonin synthesis and release is associated with an increase in their aggressive conduct. While serotonin plays an important role in aggression, it is not the only factor that bears an influence on this behaviour. The dopaminergic and noradrenaline systems may also act as facilitators of aggressive behaviour.

> Aggression is strongly influenced by social factors, such as an individual's status within its group, and a dog's past experiences.

HORMONES

Hormones also play an important part in controlling conducts associated with aggression. The endocrine and central nervous systems are closely interrelated, which means hormone levels are strictly regulated through feedback systems. A single hormone can in fact produce different and complex effects. What is more, the levels of such a hormone can influence those of other hormones and, by the same token, be influenced by yet more hormones due to complicated, feedback-controlled systems.

Just as hormones have an effect on agonistic behaviour, aggressiveness can cause changes in hormone levels. Furthermore, the actual effects of the hormones may be influenced by the individual's social context.

The hormones that influence aggressive behaviour in vertebrates, each inducing different reactions, are:
- Corticotropin: inhibits aggression.
- Catecholamines: these neurohormones, including dopamine, epinephrine (adrenaline), and norepinephrine (noradrenaline), fulfil an important function in the stress response.
- Glucocorticoids: involved in submissive responses.
- Reproductive hormones: most fights between males are due to competition for access to females. However, more fights occur between females competing for resources and food, or defending their litters, as prolactin (a hormone secreted by lactating mothers) increases aggressiveness.

Yet females tend to be less aggressive than males, as hormones involved in ovulation reduce aggression (progesterone).

➤ Sex hormones: androgens cause an increase in offensive aggression, but do not have any effect on defensive aggression. Having said that, there is no clear evidence of a correlation between high androgen plasma levels and aggressiveness, so male hormones are believed to have an organisational rather than excitatory effect on intrasexual and competitive aggression (i.e., offensive aggression).

CLASSIFICATION OF AGGRESSIVE BEHAVIOUR IN PET DOGS

To understand the concept of aggressiveness, we need to learn about the different means of classifying aggression.

BASED ON NERVE STRUCTURES

When certain parts of the brain are stimulated, it gives rise to violent or aggressive conduct regardless of the situation, context, or the individual's previous experiences. Drawing on these findings, aggressive behaviour has been classified as:

➤ **Affective aggression.** This type of aggression is regulated by the amygdaloid body and frontal cortex with the participation of serotonergic, cholinergic, and catecholaminergic transmitters. It encompasses offensive and defensive aggression, while dogs exhibiting the behaviour find it an aversive and unpleasant action. Affective aggression is characterised by a change in temperament and observable sympathetic activation (piloerection, mydriasis, etc.).

➤ **Nonaffective or predatory aggression.** This conduct originates in the hypothalamus and acetylcholine is the main neurotransmitter involved in its control. In this sort of aggression, the animal experiences positive reinforcement. It is triggered by its prey's movement or the perception of its vicinity. Nonaffective aggression prompts only a slight change in the animal's character and it is an innate, automatic response.

BASED ON THE SITUATION OR STIMULUS THAT ELICITS THE AGGRESSION

Different types of aggression have been observed between animals according to the situation or stimulus that elicits it:

- **Predatory aggression:** caused by the presence of a natural quarry.
- Antipredatory aggression: triggered by the presence of a predator.
- **Territorial aggression:** to defend an individual's domain from an intruder.
- **Dominance aggression:** exhibited when an individual's social rank is challenged or because it wants to gain access to a critical resource.
- **Maternal aggression:** provoked by the proximity of any agent that represents a threat to a mother's litter.
- **Weaning aggression:** prompted by the offspring's growing independence; parents will threaten or even gently attack their young.
- **Disciplinary parental aggression:** due to various stimuli such as out-of-hours breastfeeding, rough or excessively long games, distancing, and so on.
- **Sexual aggression:** induced by the same stimuli that trigger sexual behaviours.
- **Intermale aggression:** resulting from the presence of another male competitor.
- **Fear aggression:** in response to confinement or feeling cornered and unable to escape, or the presence of a threatening agent.

MODIFIED MOYER'S CLASSIFICATION

Kenneth E. Moyer developed a classification of aggressive behaviours based on the stimulus or causal situation that triggers the aggressive response. Many authors still use Moyer's classification to this day.

- **Dominance aggression**
- **Intraspecific aggression:** between individuals of the same species (both between males and between females)
- **Interspecific aggression:** between individuals from different species
- **Predatory aggression**
- **Pain aggression**
- **Instrumental aggression**
- **Fear aggression**
- **Territorial aggression**
- **Maternal aggression**
- **Redirected aggression**
- **Aggression secondary to pathophysiological changes**

SOCIOPATHIES

Other authors, however, with an alternative approach to animal behaviour do not define aggression problems according to a strict classification, but rather they refer to sociopathies and differentiate between two states:

- **Reactive state:** characterised by a regulated, organised sequence of aggression. It is considered a perfectly normal social behaviour for dogs.
- **Secondary hyperaggressive state:** characterised by the departure of elements that regulate aggression. It is considered a fully pathological state.

These authors also believe that acts of hierarchical, irritable, and territorial aggression comprise the hallmark trident of clinical signs observed in sociopathies.

AGONISTIC BEHAVIOUR

A recent development is the concept of agonistic behaviour, which alludes to:

➤ Competitive interaction between two or more individuals: this involves body gestures and displays related to fighting, including threats made through sounds, postures, and subtle facial expressions.

➤ Defensive attack: comprising aggressive behaviour, flight, submissive signals, threats, and biting.

➤ Offensive attack: includes hunting behaviour and biting.

KEY POINTS ON AGGRESSION

➤ Aggression is a multidimensional concept and can happen in various contexts.

➤ Aggressive behaviour is influenced by two factors: genetics and environment.

➤ Displays of aggressive behaviour involve the interaction of various factors: hormonal, neurological, cognitive, social, external stimuli, amongst others.

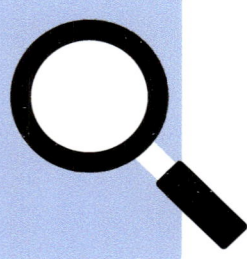

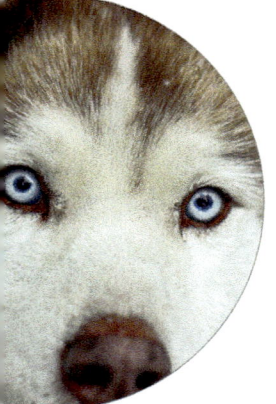

DOMINANCE AGGRESSION

Dominant or dominance aggression is the most commonplace of all aggressive behavioural disorders observed in pet dogs. This alteration is generally encountered in entire males from the age of 18 months and is more prevalent in purebreds compared to mixed-breed dogs.

The aesthetic attributes normally desired in show dogs (an erect tail, proud demeanour, and raised head) are similar to the attitudes and gestures typical of dominant animals. The dogs that win the most competitions generally tend to have more chances to reproduce, which further concentrates any genes with potentially dominant characteristics. This issue currently represents one of the main reasons for the appearance of dominance aggression (Fig. 2).

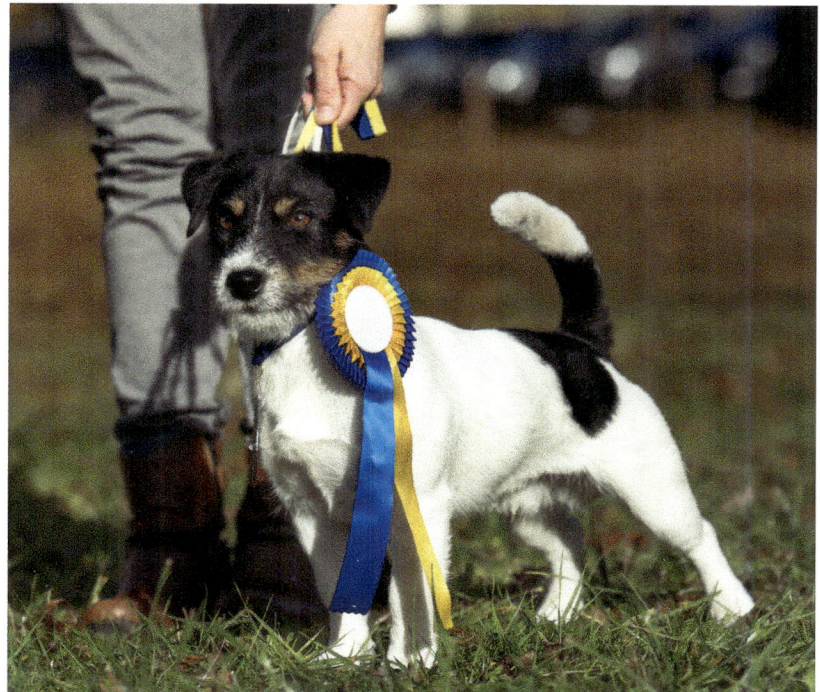

Figure 2. The search for aesthetic qualities in competitive show dogs has led to the concentration of genes with potentially dominant traits.

A dominant aggressive dog may be aggressive with one or all members of the household. Considering that the canine world is ruled by strong gestures, postures, and bodily contacts and, moreover, that dogs view their human family as members of their social group, the specific stimuli that trigger aggression derive from moments of physical contact with their owners, for example when stroking, brushing, putting the dog's collar on, and so on. Owners do not realise that these stimuli can elicit the dominant behaviour and they find it hard to understand their dog's aggressive reaction.

Dominance aggression begins when the owner allows the animal to show signs of dominance, whether due to fear or ignorance, with which the dog starts believing it is dominant and tries to subordinate its owner.

SIGNS OF DOMINANCE

Dominant animals usually emit a warning through their behaviour before resorting to direct aggression. Some tell-tale attitudes include:

➤ Pressing their head against a person's knees.
➤ Staring directly and unwaveringly at a person's eyes (Fig. 3).
➤ Standing in the owner's path and refusing to move.

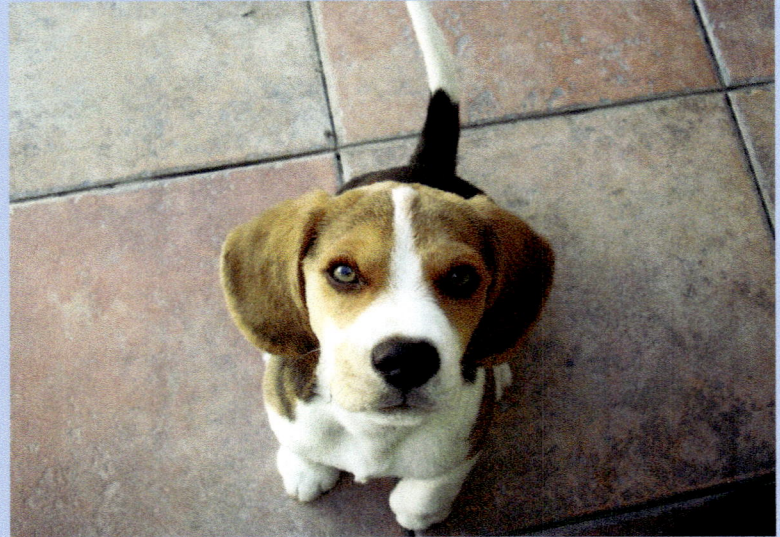

Figure 3. Dog in a dominant posture with a fixed gaze.

A permissive upbringing without any clear limits during puppyhood leads to the appearance of this alteration when the dog reaches adulthood.

DIAGNOSIS

An approximate, although not necessarily definitive, diagnosis can be made if a dog attacks someone (Fig. 4) under any of the following circumstances:

➤ When someone approaches the animal or if it is bothered while resting.

➤ When trying to protect important resources: food, a resting area, favourite items or a specific family member with whom it is very close.

➤ When it is about to be punished.

➤ If stared at for too long.

➤ When handled physically: upon being picked up, stroked, kissed, hugged, and such.

➤ When someone wants to send the dog out of the room.

➤ When a family member who lives with the dog enters the home.

Veterinary surgeons need to consider a series of points concerning the dog, its behaviour, and its everyday living environment. They need to know about the composition of the family group and possibly even their personalities. It is important to contemplate whether the household includes any children, seniors, or sick people when dealing with dominance aggression.

The vet's primary concern should be to safeguard public health, which, in this case, corresponds to the health and safety of people.

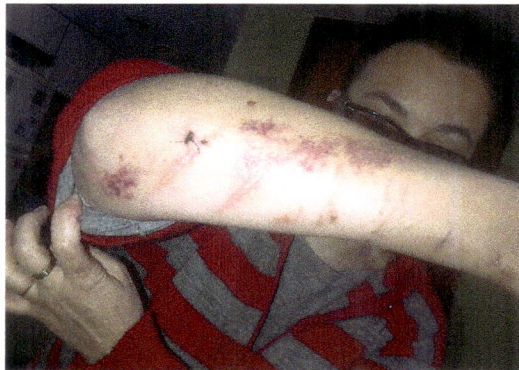

Figure 4. An owner injured by his dog.

BEHAVIOURAL DISORDERS IN DOGS

FACTORS TO CONSIDER

➤ The breed of dog.
➤ Family history.
➤ Duration the dog has been exhibiting the aggressive behaviour.
➤ The level of danger for family members.
➤ Each household member's capacity to cope with the dominant dog.

TREATMENT

In some cases, physical confrontation can reverse or curb this problem. Nevertheless, not all owners are capable of confronting their pets due to their considerable dentition and large size, especially when dealing with animals that weigh over 40 kg.

> Punishment is contraindicated in cases of dominance aggression because it will trigger an even more aggressive reaction from the dog.

➤ **Behavioural therapy:** this behaviour is very hard to modify, owners must be prepared to invest plenty of time, determination, and patience. Owners should be asked to sign a treatment authorisation stating that they are aware of the potential risks associated with behavioural therapy. It is important to stress that punishment is contraindicated when treating dominant aggressive dogs. The goals of behavioural therapy are:
  ➤ To prevent human injuries: the owner must try to avoid all attitudes which the dog could interpret as a challenge to its dominance, thus averting potentially dangerous situations.
  ➤ Invert the dog's and owner's perceptions of the hierarchical order: start with a detailed behaviour modification programme. This could include, for example, withdrawing affection and social attention when the dog shows any signs of aggression, teaching it some simple dominance exercises (e.g. sitting and receiving a reward when done correctly), or taking longer walks to use up more energy, as dogs that act

aggressively towards their owners at home might be more passive in the street because they feel less confident. Vets must convince owners that they can handle their animal.

For behavioural therapy to be effective, it is a good idea to give household members a list to remind them of the new handling guidelines, as this will guide owners when carrying out the dominance exercises through some practical sessions.

- **Drug treatment:** this mainly involves synthetic progestogens, which should always be prescribed in combination with a behaviour modification programme:
  - Synthetic progesterones: prescribe oral megestrol acetate at a dosage of 2 mg/kg/day taken orally in one or two doses, for 2 weeks. Then halve the dosage every 2 weeks, up to a maximum course of 8 weeks. Megestrol acetate reduces aggressiveness in males by lowering testosterone levels and, given its marked anxiolytic effect, it also grants owners better control over their pet while performing the behaviour modification programme. Ideally, pre- and posttreatment blood tests should be conducted since this type of medication can have some adverse side effects.
  - Benzodiazepine anxiolytics: a typical dosage for drugs such as clonazepam is 0.5–2.0 mg/kg/day taken orally and spread across two or three doses to reach and maintain a minimum safe concentration while carrying out the behaviour modification techniques. Each case should, however, be assessed on an individual basis according to the animal's and owner's personalities.

> Drug treatment is an aid to behavioural therapy in patients manifesting dominance aggression, and not the other way around.

- **Surgical treatment:** surgical castration is indicated in males, obviously, as an alternative to progesterone therapy. An advantage of castration is that it does not have the potential side effects of hormone therapy.

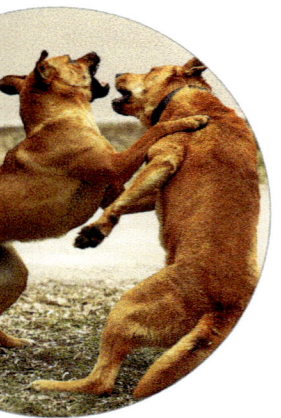

INTRASPECIFIC AND INTRASEXUAL AGGRESSION

AGGRESSION BETWEEN MALES

This behaviour is commonly observed in homes with male dogs, where aggression may be observed between cohabitants in houses with multiple males or in public spaces with males from outside the home if the patient lives alone.

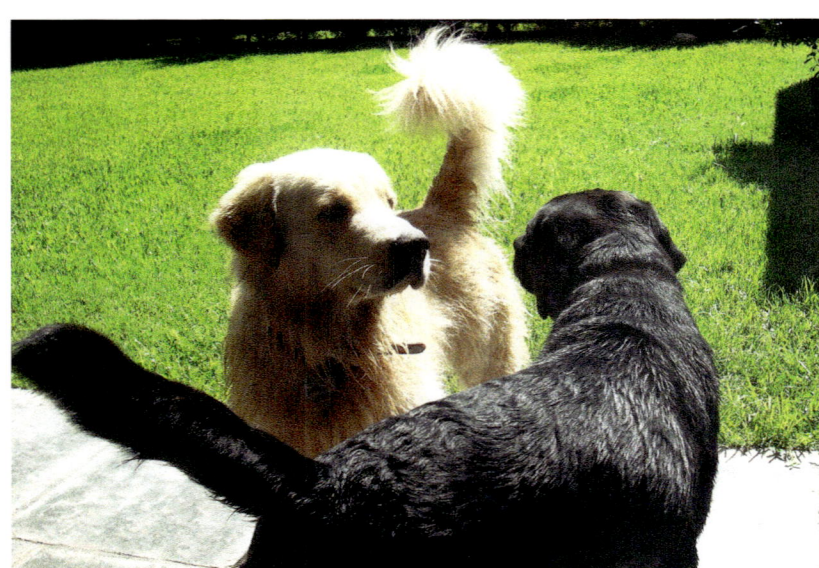

Figure 5.
Aggression between males is influenced by testosterone.

DIAGNOSIS

This behavioural disorder is observed in entire males aged 1–3 years and incidence is independent of the breed. This sort of aggression is influenced by the male hormone testosterone (Fig. 5).

TREATMENT

Both progesterone therapy and castration sharply curb this behavioural alteration. Even better outcomes can be achieved if these treatments are used in combination with counterconditioning techniques that include progressive approaches and rewards for correct behaviour.

➤ **Behavioural therapy:** owners need to exert authority over their dogs through dominance exercises. There are two main situations:
  ➤ Dogs that fight with unknown dogs: this scenario should be corrected through the owner's absolute dominance and by scolding the animal's aggressive attitude.
  ➤ Dogs that fight with others in the same household: these cases are much harder to resolve. Treatment is based on the application of counterconditioning techniques in order to inhibit the aggressive behaviour. It is often the owner who actually generates the conflict by siding with the "weaker" dog and therefore preventing the animals from establishing a natural hierarchy.

➤ **Drug treatment:** if the owner opts against castration for their dogs, a viable alternative is to give them female hormones; however, although the medication is generally effective, the same problem will resurface as soon as it is discontinued. The treatment involves hormone therapy with synthetic progesterones; 1–2 mg/kg/day of megestrol acetate, taken orally in one or two doses for 2 weeks. Then administer half the initial dosage for another 2 weeks. Progesterones produce a pronounced reduction of characteristically male attitudes and an anxiolytic effect on the brain. A blood test should be carried out before starting the hormone therapy, placing particular attention on the blood glucose level and white blood cell count.

➤ **Surgical treatment:** one treatment option is to castrate the dogs involved in the conflicts. Surgical castration reduces aggression between males in 62 % of cases.

AGGRESSION BETWEEN FEMALES

In this case, the origin lies in the failure to establish a hierarchical order between the females in the household (Fig. 6).

The owner must have an authoritative command over the female dogs that fight to be able to constrain their desire for confrontation. However, the females will probably start fighting again when the owner is absent, so they should be separated whenever the owner is not around to control them.

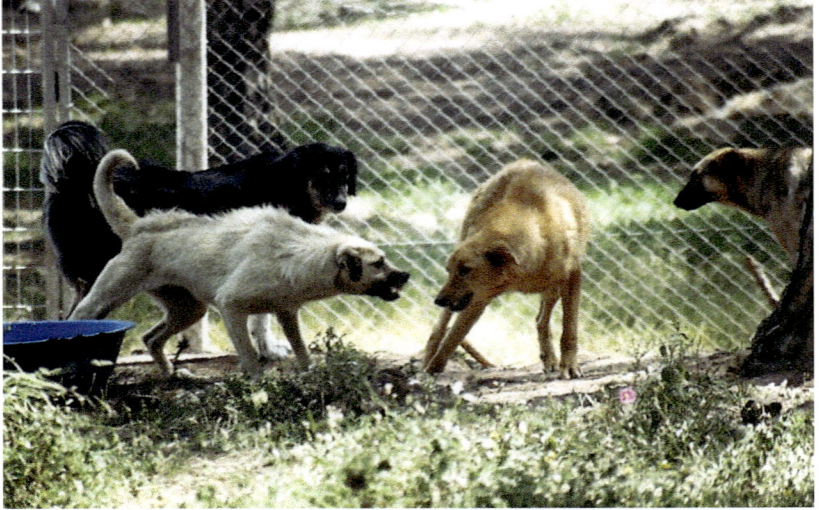

Figure 6. A lack of hierarchical order between female dogs that live together leads to intrasexual aggression.

DIAGNOSIS

It occurs in both intact and castrated females aged 1–3 years, but older dogs can also exhibit the behaviour. Breed does not have any bearing on the incidence.

> This disorder is much harder to resolve than aggression between males, as hormones bear very little influence.

TREATMENT

➤ **Behavioural therapy:** the only treatment indicated for aggression between females is resocialisation using behavioural modification techniques.

➤ **Surgical treatment:** castration does not generally have any positive effects, except for the case of fights that occur when females are in oestrous. Castration is, therefore, contraindicated, since removing the source of female hormones would increase the level of aggression between females.

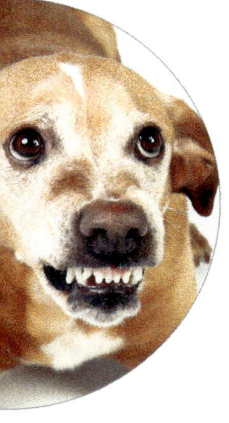

FEAR AGGRESSION

This develops in insecure and timid dogs. These dogs feel cornered and bite when approached by an unknown individual of any species. In general, their bites are not too serious, as they lack conviction. Their only objective is to drive away the stimulus causing their fear. Fear aggression is often the product of traumatic experiences, for example, owners who are excessively strict or violent when interacting with their dog. These animals should be handled without rushing in, as they require behavioural therapy and medication to overcome their phobias.

DIAGNOSIS

The incidence is the same in intact or castrated males and females regardless of age or breed. It can be diagnosed through direct observation of the classic fear posture (slightly cowered, tail between the legs, and ears turned down, Fig. 7) and based on information from the anamnesis.

TREATMENT

➤ **Behavioural therapy:** the correct treatment is to desensitise the animal. Punishment is contraindicated as a means of controlling dogs with fear aggression; it is essential that owners understand the need to change how they handle their dog.

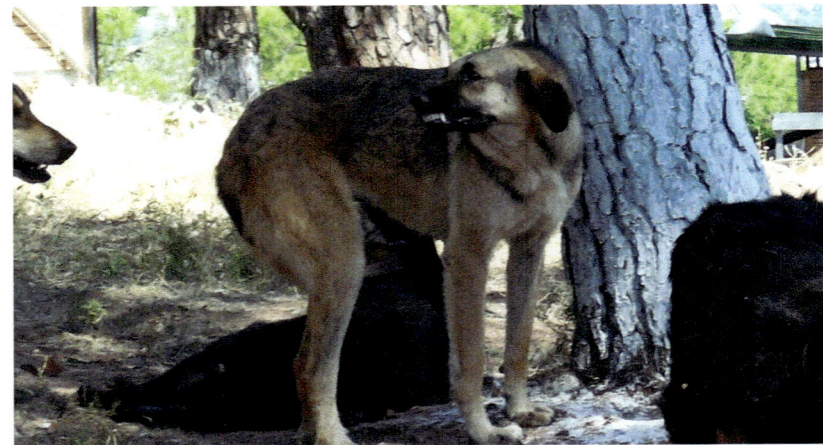

Figure 7. The typical fear posture is a slightly cowered position, with the tail between the legs, and ears turned down.

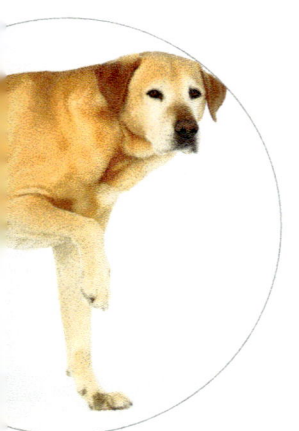

➤ **Drug treatment:** antiphobic drugs are used to treat this type of aggression. The most used option is clonazepam at similar dosages to those indicated to treat other types of behavioural disorders related to fear and phobias. An indicative dosage is 0.5–2.0 mg/kg/day taken orally and spread over two or three doses. The diagnosis must be accurate, as dosages for psychoactive drugs are generally only for guidance. This sort of treatment, unlike others, depends heavily on individual patient idiosyncrasies in order to achieve the desired effect. Progesterone therapy is not effective in fear aggression.

PAIN AGGRESSION

Pain aggression is a protective action for the animal, as it is used as a means of defence. Be that as it may, we cannot tolerate an animal that bites when subject to certain actions such as treating a wound or cleaning its ears. This behaviour can be warded off by getting dogs used to these handling activities while they are still puppies, even though they might be a little painful.

DIAGNOSIS

The incidence of pain aggression is independent of age, sex, and breed.

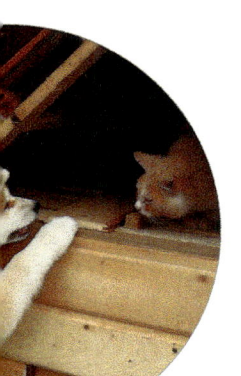

TREATMENT

➤ **Behavioural therapy:** punishment is contraindicated; the correct approach is the use of counterconditioning techniques, desensitisation, and rewards for appropriate behaviour. In addition, owners must establish themselves as the absolute leaders during the dog's upbringing.

PREDATORY AGGRESSION

This is aggression directed towards whatever the dog sees as prey. A typical example is dogs that chase cyclists, runners, or cats (Fig. 8). In these situations, the dog is at serious risk of suffering or causing an accident in the public highway. During the anamnesis, owners usually tell the story of an obedient, gentle dog which, as soon as it sees a cat, starts chasing its 'prey' without heeding commands. Owners may think that they rule over their dogs, but they need to understand and accept that it is not the case.

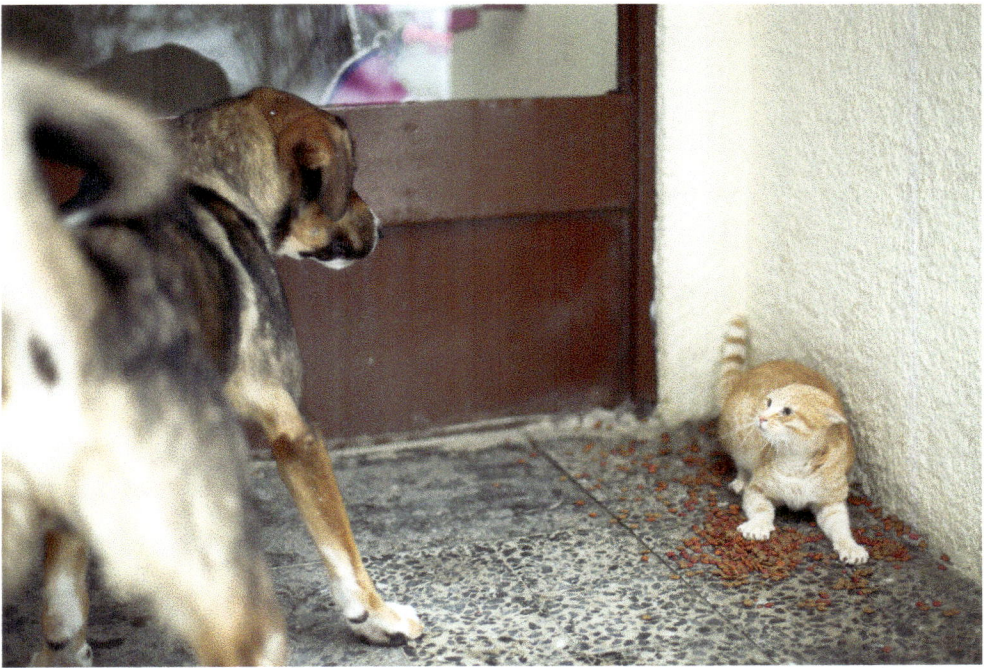

Figure 8. Dogs that chase cats are one example of predatory aggression.

DIAGNOSIS

This type of aggression disorder is more common among breeds with a strong hunting or predatory instinct. The diagnosis is based on information gleaned from the anamnesis.

> Ultimately, predatory aggression underlines a lack of leadership and control from the dog's owner.

TREATMENT

➤ **Behavioural therapy:** predatory aggression is treated with behaviour modification techniques and by ensuring the owner has total dominance over their dog.

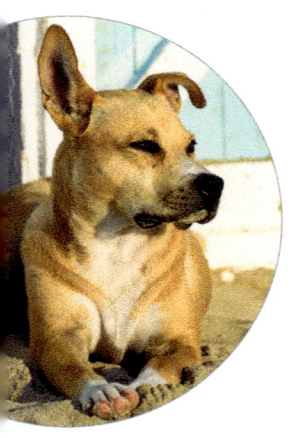

TERRITORIAL AGGRESSION

Territorial aggression is a normal conduct in dogs. This behaviour is often desired and reinforced by owners who want their pets to act as guard dogs. However, they tend to become too aggressive and the situation develops into a problem when dogs start trying to attack visitors, postal workers, passers-by, and so on (Fig. 9).

This situation is best avoided by training dogs while young and taking care not to promote territorial aggression as they will naturally exhibit the behaviour when older.

DIAGNOSIS

Territorial aggression first manifests at 8–9 months and can be observed in both males and females. Breed does not have a significant bearing on incidence, although the problem is evidently more pronounced in large breeds.

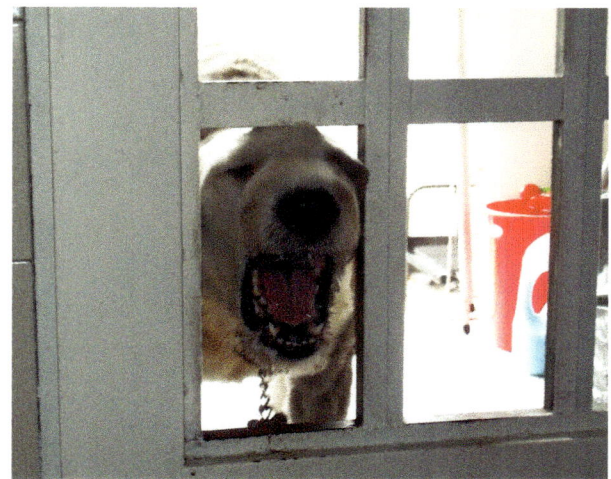

Figure 9. Territorial aggression is a normal behaviour in dogs, but it should not be encouraged to reach excessive levels.

TREATMENT

➤ **Behavioural therapy:** counterconditioning is used to train dogs to stop attacking other individuals. This can only be achieved while the owner is present.

➤ **Drug treatment:** hormone therapies can be used to treat territorial aggression.

➤ **Surgical treatment:** castration is only carried out in males. The efficacy depends on the dog's age when castrated and the owner's ability to exert leadership.

MATERNAL AGGRESSION

This behaviour is displayed by mothers with newborn pups and is influenced by hormone levels. It generally starts to disappear 1 month after parturition. The relationship between the female dog and its owners will determine whether or not she exhibits this behaviour. Ideally, owners should take precautions, such as disturbing the mother as little as possible, and if the behaviour needs to be corrected immediately, apply positive reinforcement of the desired behaviour. They should not resort to punishment. It is vital that owners understand they must prevent anyone from annoying female dogs when they are with their pups.

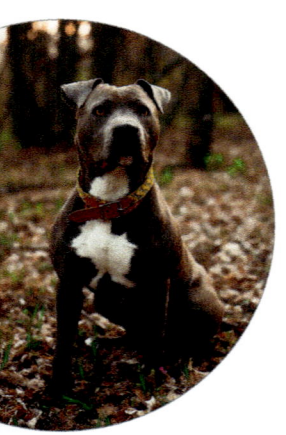

AGGRESSION DUE TO PATHOPHYSIOLOGICAL CONDITIONS

In this case the aggressive behaviour is due to a neurological disorder, which is secondary to a physicochemical clinical alteration. There is a myriad of underlying anatomico-physiological diseases that can contribute to the onset of a behavioural disorder in pet dogs. Naturally, this complication requires a strictly medical resolution since the abnormal behaviour is the result of a clinical problem. In most cases, and after resolving the underlying clinical issue, patients will continue to exhibit the behavioural alteration because they have been conditioned to act in such a manner, so behavioural therapy is also indicated to address the problem successfully.

DIAGNOSIS

A precise diagnosis can only be made after completing all the necessary veterinary examinations. Neurological and hormonal diseases are responsible for most of the cases of aggression due to pathophysiological causes. It is important to focus on aggressive behaviour due to pain caused by a clinical condition, such as an osteoarticular disease, particularly in elderly dogs.

In aggression due to pathophysiological conditions, the underlying clinical disease is the main cause of the aggressive behaviour. Of all the hormonal conditions to stimulate aggression in dogs, thyroid disorders, particularly hypothyroidism, are some of the most frequently observed in clinical practice.

Furthermore, many behavioural problems can derive from past or current infections of the nervous system, for example distemper, or biochemical abnormalities thereof (genetic mutations in brain neurotransmitters). In practice, the observation of excessive, uncontrolled aggression is often due to subclinical psychomotor epilepsy, in which case the dog's electro-encephalogram (EEG) will have an epileptogenic focus. This focus is not intense enough to trigger convulsions, but it will precipitate clearly aggressive behaviour. It results in unpredictable, idiopathic, and spontaneous attacks on people, animals, or even objects.

> The prognosis can range from guarded to severe due to the potential danger this behavioural disorder represents for third parties.

TREATMENT

➤ **Drug treatment:** treatment to resolve or improve the underlying illness will depend on the clinical diagnosis thereof. Possible pharmacological treatments include all drugs indicated for the clinical treatment of the diagnosed disease (antiepileptic drugs, hormone replacement therapies, etc.).

ANNEX
GUIDELINES FOR OWNERS

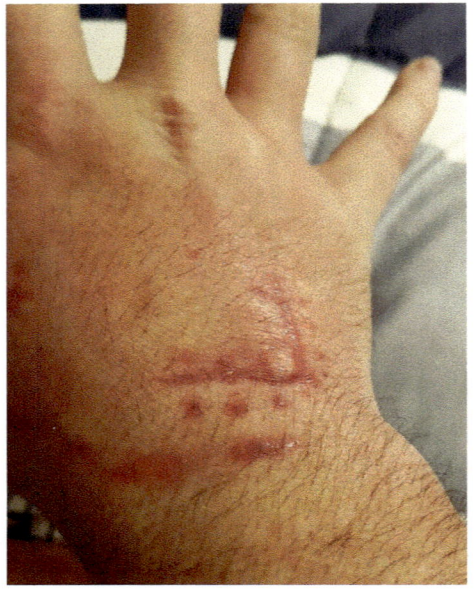

Figure 10. Owner bitten by their own dog.

Aggression in dogs is a very common animal behavioural problem and mainly derives from inappropriate handling by the dog's owners (Fig. 10). Logically, the traits inherent to each breed influence this behaviour, but breed is not a determining factor.

Once the aggressive behaviour has been correctly diagnosed, it should be treated in a collaborative process between the vet and the dog's owner. Besides the appropriate drug therapy or surgical treatment, behavioural therapy is always necessary to address the problem and this relies on proactive participation from the owners.

AIMS OF BEHAVIOURAL THERAPY

➤ To revert the dominance–subordination relationship that exists between the animal and its owner.
➤ To train the dog to allow people or other animals in its vicinity without acting aggressively.
➤ To condition the dog to react with nonaggressive conducts when situations that normally stimulate its aggression arise.

Therapy is based on three essential pillars:

➤ Drug therapy or surgery, where appropriate.

➤ Correct treatment by those who live with the aggressive dog, following the indications given during the consultation.

➤ Resocialisation through the application of dominance exercises, counterconditioning techniques, and so on, to be conducted by the owner with follow-up and advice from a veterinary professional.

Since dogs with an aggression-related behavioural disorder represent a potential danger to others, their owners must be aware of their legal responsibilities and, similarly, familiar with all the implications of the treatment and the risks of living with dogs presenting such problems.

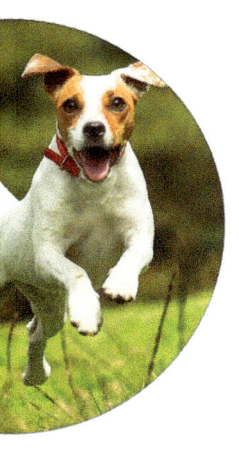

HOW TO BE A DOG'S LEADER

When roughly 6 months old, dogs enter into an adolescent stage that lasts until the age of about 18 months. Dogs do not obey even the most straightforward orders during this adolescent stage. Throughout this period, young dogs try to position themselves within the hierarchy of their social group.

Owners must endeavour to reinforce their position as leader while dogs are adolescents. Some recommendations to help them with this include:

➤ Practise dominance exercises.

➤ Always talk to the dog with a calm, nonthreatening voice.

➤ Take the dog for regular walks.

➤ Carefully and gently hold the dog's mouth closed; this a dominant gesture understood by the adolescent dog that will help consolidate the owner's position of ascendancy.

➤ Do not tolerate mounting behaviour, particularly with children.

➤ Say "no" with a stern, cutting tone, but without shouting or getting angry with the dog.

The first signs of aggression should be quashed using appropriate measures as soon as they appear, since it is much harder to correct a well-established undesired behaviour than to prevent it from the outset.

All family members must clearly understand that the dog occupies the lowest echelon in the hierarchy, because any dog which believes it is above a family member may develop serious aggression-related behavioural problems, especially males.

> An excellent mantra to apply when teaching dogs is the three Ps
> – practice, patience, and perseverance.

Dogs that have been subjected to violence since they were puppies tend to suffer anxiety, may start biting others when afraid, and could lose trust in humans, so the use of force should be completely discouraged. Dogs in general, and above all males, can misinterpret physical affection for gestures that signal their owners' subordination to them; therefore, owners should minimise any typically human displays of affection. Stronger leadership can be achieved through the use of simple orders, consistency in day-to-day treatment, respect, and affection.

HOW TO COPE WITH A DOMINANCE PROBLEM

- ➤ Withhold the dog's social attention: ignore the animal and try to reduce physical contact with it during the course of the treatment.
- ➤ Limit any contact with the dog to when it obeys an order or assumes a position of obedience. Owners should not be concerned with the dog and its actions.
- ➤ Increase the animal's level of physical activity with more walks; always use a collar and lead.
- ➤ Practise the dominance exercises.

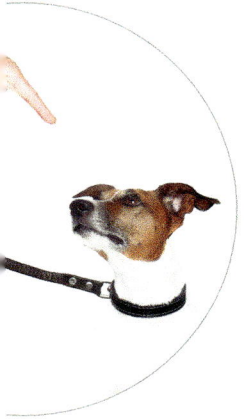

DOMINANCE EXERCISES

This subsection explains four minimal and essential dominance exercises to help attain basic control over a dog. A choke collar should be used in all cases. There are three main types: chains, cord, or leather. We generally recommend collars made of cord with a thickness that corresponds to the dog's atlantoaxial notch. The most popular choice is a 6 or 8 mm thick, cord choke collar. Above all, they must not cause the dog trauma or endanger their physical wellbeing, and they must be the right size for the dog. Choke collars should not be used as a punishment, but instead as a means of controlling the dog.

SITTING POSITION

The "sit" exercise is easily achieved; place the choke collar in the correct position and pull the lead upwards. At the same time, use your free hand to firmly and constantly press the dog's rump downwards, taking care to avoid sudden movements, while saying "sit" in a firm tone, but without ever shouting.

WALKING TO HEEL

The walking to heel exercise (Fig. 11) involves walking the dog with the choke collar in the correct position but without tightening it too much; when the dog tries to get ahead of the owner, they should give a small backward tug on the lead while repeating the command "heel". This should be done with a strong, firm voice, but without shouting.

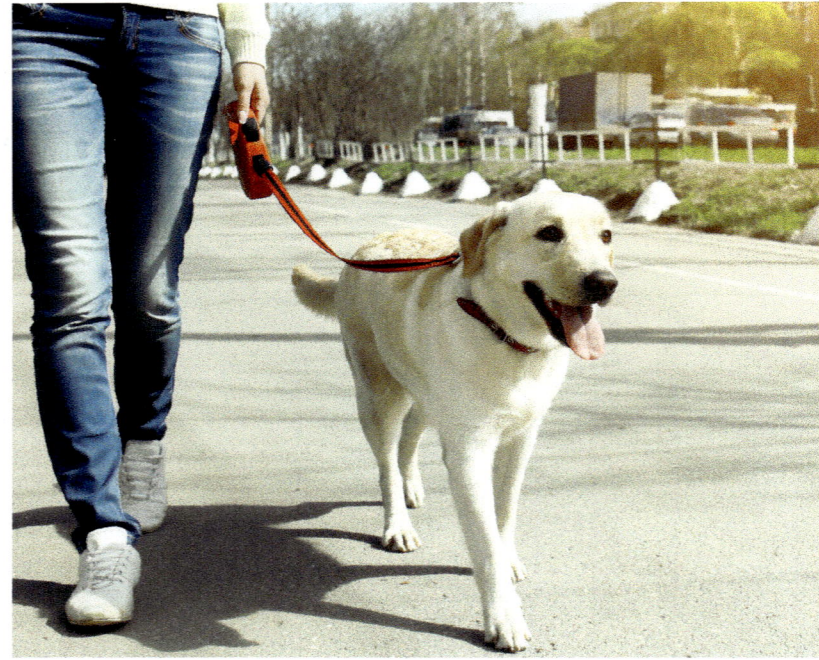

Figure 11.
Walking to heel
exercise.

TRAINING THE ORDER TO STOP AN ACTION

This involves teaching the dog that when its owner says a certain word, then it must stop whatever it is doing at that given moment. The order should only ever be used when the animal is carrying out an undesired action and never in any other situation.

Owners can start teaching this command while walking in the street with the dog well-controlled on its lead. At some point, the animal will want to pull in another direction or stop to smell something. At that very instant, the owner should tug on the lead and say the order "stop", then adjust the dog into the correct position and make it sit. Inside the home, if the animal is about to do something wrong, the owner should firmly give the order to stop.

Although at first the dog may not understand the order, it will quickly associate the word with its desired meaning. It is fundamental that the order is always used whenever a conflictive situation arises and that everyone in the household uses it consistently under the same circumstances. Another consideration is that walks should be a pleasurable act for the dog, so periods of training should be intercalated with relaxing, enjoyable moments.

POSITIVE REINFORCEMENT OF OBEDIENCE

Positive reinforcement of obedient behaviour means rewarding dogs when they comply with orders. It can be applied through congratulations and affectionate pats, but while avoiding excessive stroking. Using food as a reward would be ill-advised, as it could sow the seeds for a future compulsive eating behaviour (Fig. 12).

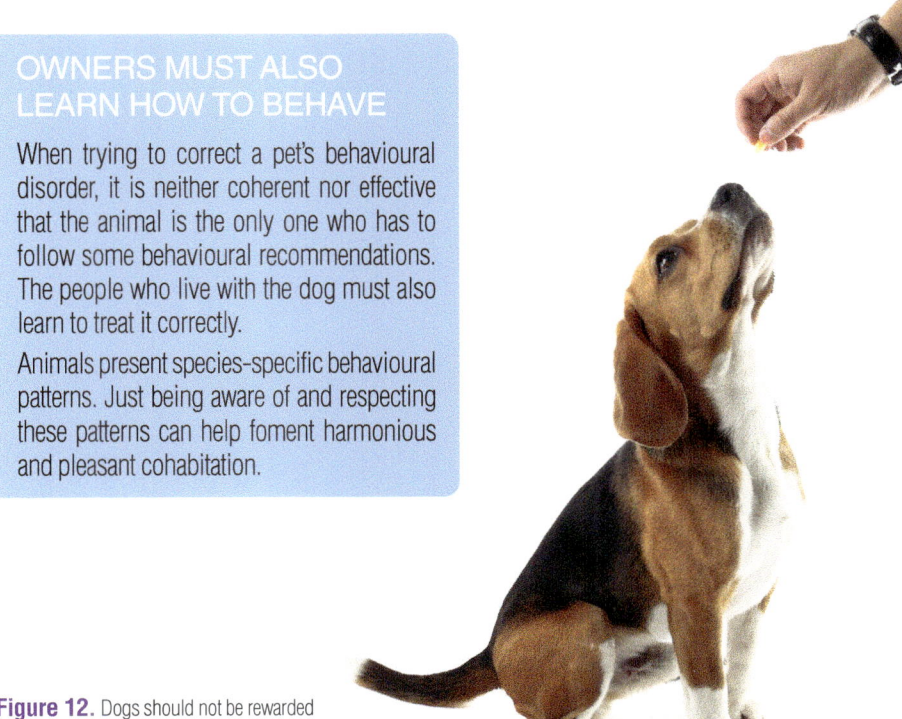

OWNERS MUST ALSO LEARN HOW TO BEHAVE

When trying to correct a pet's behavioural disorder, it is neither coherent nor effective that the animal is the only one who has to follow some behavioural recommendations. The people who live with the dog must also learn to treat it correctly.

Animals present species-specific behavioural patterns. Just being aware of and respecting these patterns can help foment harmonious and pleasant cohabitation.

Figure 12. Dogs should not be rewarded with food, otherwise they could develop compulsive eating disorders in the future.

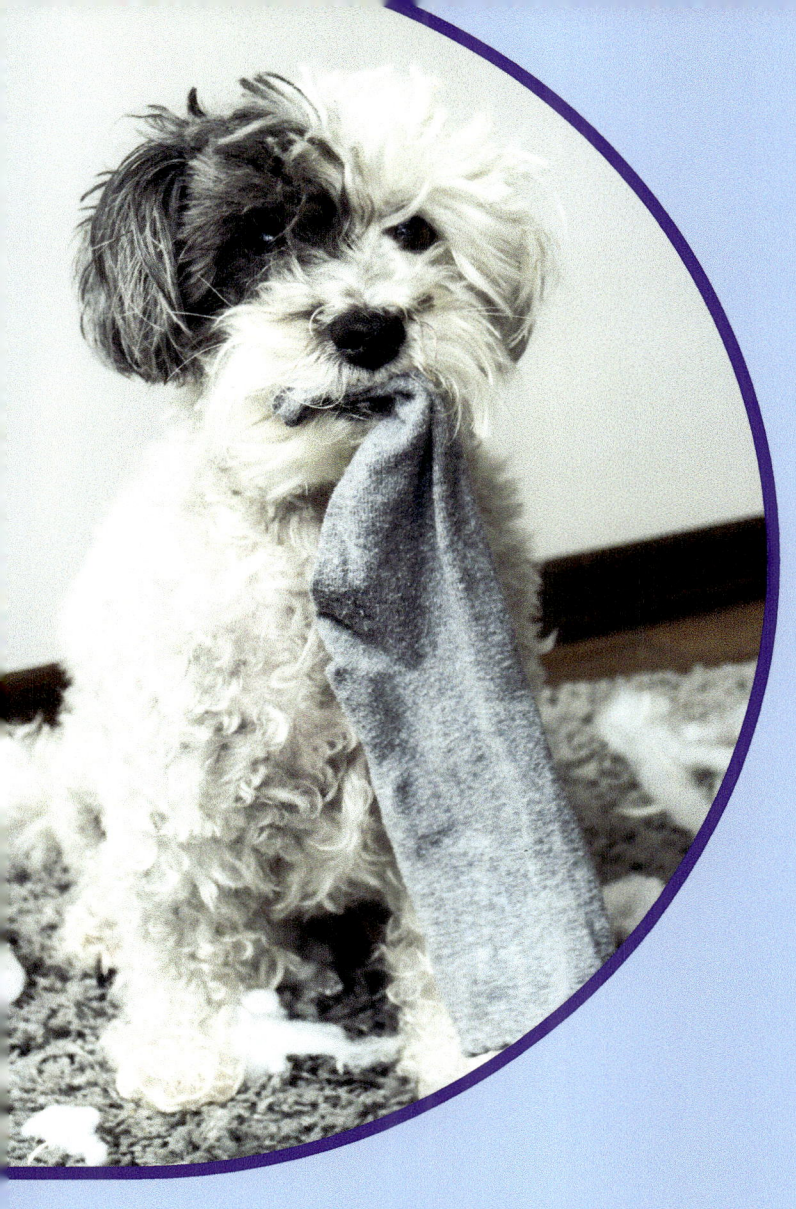

DISORDERS ASSOCIATED WITH ANXIETY AND STRESS

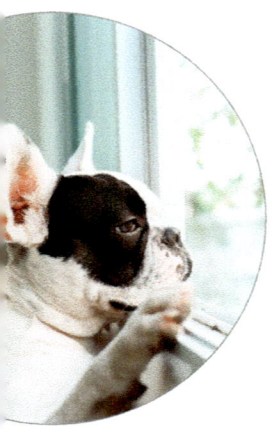

INTRODUCTION

Behavioural problems related to anxiety and stress are very common among pets, particularly dogs. Obviously, this is influenced by each animal's characteristics, as some animals are more predisposed to anxious behaviour in certain environmental or emotional situations than others.

Anxiety is defined as a state of psychophysical distress characterised by confusion or restlessness, and insecurity or fear of a perceived immediate threat.

Stress is an individual's physiological response to any of its given stressors.

STRESSORS

The main stressors for household pets are:

➤ Physical: adverse environmental conditions (too cold, hot, noisy, etc.), too much or too little (sedentary) physical activity, pain and somatic illnesses (abuse or diseases), and so on.

➤ Social: excessively idle (boredom), reduced living space, alienation from the social group or changes to the components of the group, sudden habitat changes (move to a new home or alterations to the dog's space), amongst others.

In many cases, severe anxiety leads to compulsive and repetitive behaviours (constant leg licking, tail chasing, digging holes in the garden, etc.), which develop into habits, and eventually the animal will exhibit stereotyped behaviours.

TREATMENT

The generic treatment of behavioural disorders associated with anxiety and stress consists of behavioural therapy and pharmacological treatment.

BEHAVIOURAL THERAPY

The aims of behavioural therapy in the treatment of anxiety disorders focus on teaching the owner to manage the dog's states of anxiety and conditioning the dog not to engage in anxious behavioural patterns in the presence of certain stimuli. To this end, it helps to follow a series of recommendations:

➤ Avoid stimulating anxious behaviour by stroking the dog or through consenting actions (e.g. giving it food) when it becomes nervous or restless. Anxious behaviour should instead be ignored as much as possible.

➤ Increase the dog's activity levels through regular walks. Physical activity goes a long way towards resolving the disorder, as it is the most effective naturally occurring anxiolytic.

➤ Allow the dog to satisfy its species-specific behavioural needs.

> Physically impeding the compulsive behaviour is not the correct treatment for this disorder.

Professional treatment of these cases should involve identifying and correcting the stimulus that triggers the patient's conflict. Dogs should neither be punished nor physically restrained when displaying the stereotyped behaviour.

DRUG TREATMENT

The choice of psychoactive drug depends on the patient's idiosyncrasies, so all dosages are indicative and should be assessed and adjusted accordingly. The aim should be to give each patient their own tailored minimum effective dosage.

LOW-POTENCY NEUROLEPTICS

The most used neuroleptic is chlorpromazine at a dosage of 25–50 mg/animal/day taken orally in three doses. It can inhibit learning and produce anticholinergic and cardiovascular side effects. Furthermore, underdosing may trigger hyperreflexia which could, in turn, give rise to a sudden aggressive reaction.

BENZODIAZEPINE DERIVATIVE ANXIOLYTICS

The main examples are diazepam, lorazepam, and clonazepam, which are indicated to treat panic attacks or phobias at dosages of 0.5–2.0 mg/kg /day taken orally in 2-3 doses. Alprazolam at a regimen of 0.25–2.0 mg/kg/day given in two or three doses is also recommended for phobias. Of all the benzodiazepine derivatives, bromazepam has the strongest anxiolytic effect at a recommended dosage range of 0.5–2.0 mg/kg/day spread over two or three oral doses. They act by blocking GABA receptors in the central nervous system and, following prolonged treatment (which is rarely needed for animals), their main potential side effects are hepatotoxicity, nephrotoxicity, and dependence. Lorazepam and oxazepam are biotransformed in the liver by conjugation, rather than oxidation, so they pose less risk in dogs with liver disorders.

TRICYCLIC ANTIDEPRESSANTS

The two main drugs in this group are amitriptyline and clomipramine. Both are tertiary amines with a long half-life, and they cause muscarinic side effects (dry mucosae, urinary retention, and constipation) and weight gain as an antihistaminic side effect. An indicative dosage for this pharmacological group is 1–3 mg/kg/day by mouth.

SELECTIVE SEROTONIN REUPTAKE INHIBITORS (SSRIS)

The most used are fluoxetine, paroxetine, sertraline, and citalopram, which belongs to a more selective group with fewer effects on other organ systems. All are well tolerated, and their primary side effects are gastrointestinal problems (anorexia, nausea, and diarrhoea) and decreased libido, which could represent an advantage in certain behavioural alterations. Their half-life is 25 hours, so they can be given orally once a day. The recommended dosage is 0.5–1.0 mg/kg/day.

AZAPIRONES

The main example of this group is buspirone, which was the first nonsedative anxiolytic agent ever developed and has been used extensively in human psychiatry. Its mechanism of action blocks the pre- and postsynaptic serotonin-1A receptors, thereby regulating serotonin activity as well as acting as a dopamine agonist. It does not have any muscle relaxant, sedative, or anticonvulsant effects. The recommended dosage is 2.5–10.0 mg/dog split over two daily oral doses, as the half-life is approximately 14 hours.

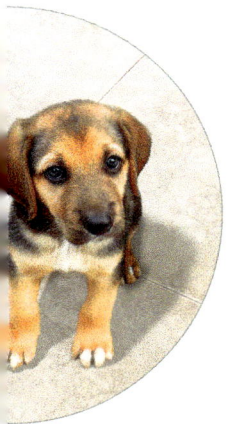

SEPARATION ANXIETY

Separation anxiety is a disorder in which the animal, when left alone, feels a lot of anxiety that it channels through the destruction of clothes or furniture, inappropriate eliminations, or, more often than not, by howling and barking, sometimes very intensely and incessantly.

DIAGNOSIS

This problem is diagnosed through the anamnesis and observations of the dog's behaviour and its relationship with its owners. The body of data in the literature does not reveal a specific predisposition according to breed, sex, or age, although it is more common among small, female, young/adult dogs.

The main signs of this problem are barking and howling whenever the dog is left alone, the elimination of urine and faeces near doors and windows, and, in the severest cases, the destruction of objects, including very large ones (Figs. 1 and 2). Animals with separation anxiety also greet their owners with exaggerated enthusiasm when they return home.

During the consultation, vets can often notice an excessive reciprocal attachment between dogs and their owners. Owners can sometimes unwittingly reinforce this anxiety by trying to explain to the dog that it will be left alone for a few hours, which provokes anxiety before the owner has even gone. What is more, owners frequently greet their dogs with too much exuberance when they get home, which excites the animal and fossilises its perception of a huge difference between being alone and with its owner.

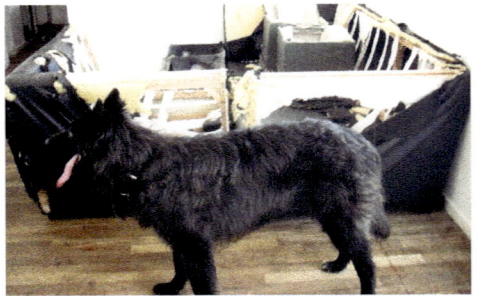
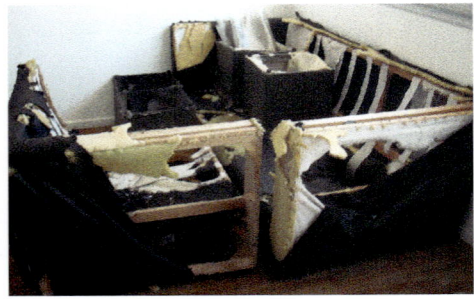

Figure 1. A sofa destroyed by a dog with separation anxiety.

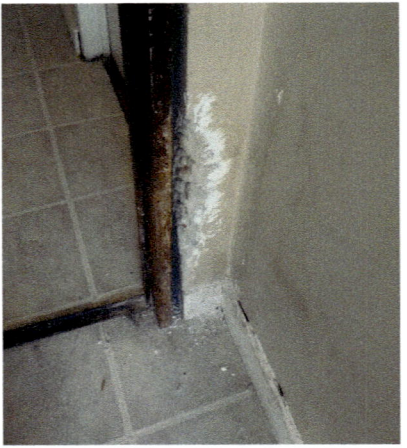
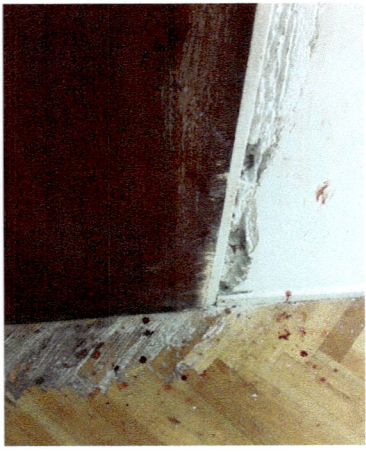

Figure 2. Dogs with separation anxiety can be very destructive when left alone.

> Before reaching a behavioural diagnosis, it is important to rule out any clinical alterations that could be causing the dog's abnormal behaviour.

TREATMENT

- ➤ **Behavioural therapy:** the treatment objective is to accustom the dog to spending time alone without the situation generating a state of agitation, anxiety, or stress. To achieve this, owners should follow a series of recommendations:
  - ➤ Increase the dog's level of physical activity.
  - ➤ Use a transitional object that is only with the dog when it is alone; as soon as a member of the family gets home, they should remove the object and place it out of sight.
  - ➤ Use food puzzle toys to hide treats and keep the dog entertained while alone.
  - ➤ It is advisable to leave the dog in an enclosed area compatible with its size (from a transport cage to a closed room where it cannot do any damage), but always with a toy. The larger the space and the more objects within reach, the greater the dog's anxiety. Before doing this, while owners are at home, they should habituate their dog to spending time in the cage without showing any signs of anxiety (groaning, whining, barking, trying to escape, destructive behaviour, etc.). If it proves impossible to train the dog to stay in the cage, it must be taught to sit and relax in a certain location in the home.
  - ➤ Desensitise the dog to the signals that precede the owner's departure (e.g. picking up keys, putting shoes on, etc.). This is achieved by doing these actions randomly a few times a day when they do not intend to leave the house, always at an intensity the dog can tolerate without provoking evident anxiety.
  - ➤ Withdraw social attention in order to gradually foster detachment, but without stimulating anxiety. Whenever the owner leaves or returns home, they should ignore their dog for 5–10 minutes.

> It is crucial for owners to avoid reinforcing their dog's anxious behaviour and that they achieve some degree of detachment when they are together.

➤ Schedule a programme of outings that consists of leaving the dog alone for short, controlled periods, which are gradually increased while alternating shorter and longer spells. It should include at least two outings a day, adhering to the above guidelines (ignoring the dog when leaving and returning home, refraining from any contact until it has calmed down, etc.). The programme has been completed successfully when the dog manages to remain calm for a period similar to the owner's regular absences.

➤ Punishment is totally contraindicated as it only aggravates the problem.

➤ **Drug treatment**
   ➤ Bromazepam: 0.5–2.0 mg/kg/day in 2–3 doses, orally.

> **PREVENTION**
>
> To prevent separation anxiety from developing, owners should give puppies time alone as soon as they arrive at their new home. Avoid giving them too much attention during the daytime and take them for walks to socialise with other dogs, puppies, and members of other species.

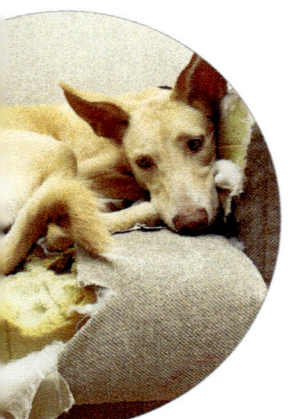

ANXIETY SYNDROME

This syndrome is a state of anxiety exacerbated by an environmental stressor. The problem stems from an unfavourable environment, with very little physical activity and a lethargic lifestyle, which can cause dogs to channel their accumulated energy into behaviours that are incompatible with cohabiting with humans. They start to break objects and display disagreeable conducts (Fig. 3), which can drive owners to isolate them from the family group (Fig. 4), and some breeds of dog may also exhibit signs of aggression towards certain family members. Social isolation, in addition to the languor and lack of exercise, can induce the animal to adopt compulsive behaviours (constant leg licking, tail chasing, digging holes in the garden, etc.) or act more aggressively toward its owners during social interactions. When this compulsive behaviour persists over time, it can develop into a compulsive syndrome and the patient may ultimately cause itself serious physical injuries. Additionally, owners tend to unintentionally reinforce the behaviour (Fig. 5).

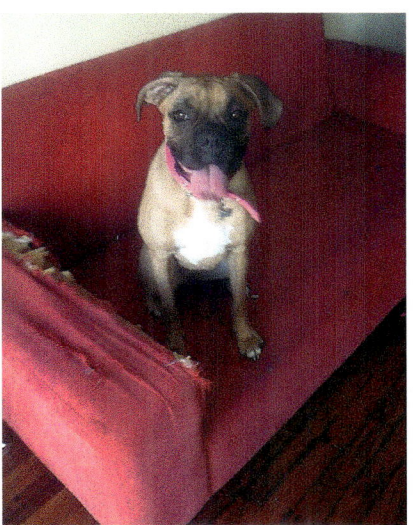

◄ **Figure 3.** An anxious dog will start to attack furniture and other items.

Figure 4. A dog isolated on a balcony away from the family group.
▼

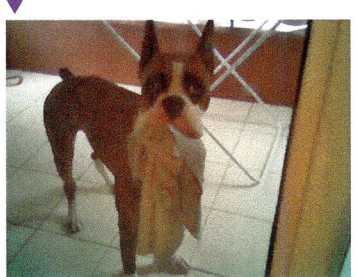

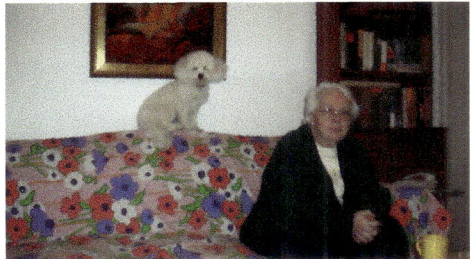

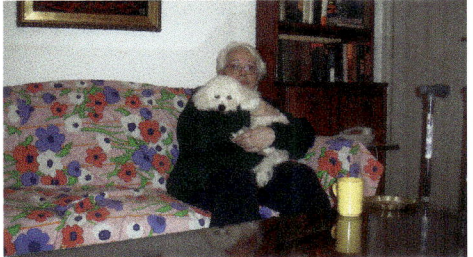

Figure 5. A lot of owners reinforce their dog's undesirable behaviour.

BEHAVIOURAL DISORDERS IN DOGS

DIAGNOSIS

Diagnosis is based on data collected from the anamnesis. It is determined by two important factors:

➤ Socialisation: poor or no socialisation due to limited contact with other puppies, adult dogs, or even other species.

➤ Breed: it generally occurs in purebred dogs and athletic biotypes (Weimaranner, Boxer, Beagle, Braco, etc.) that practise very little or no daily physical activity.

At the time of consultation, often the animal has already been isolated from the family, so the problem is compounded by the negative relation between the owners and their dog.

> ### PROGNOSIS
>
> The prognosis ranges from guarded to severe, depending primarily on the owner's personality, lifestyle, available time, and capacity to understand the cause of the problem.
>
> It is important to remember that the prognosis often also depends on the breed, biotype, and size of the animal.

TREATMENT

Treatment consists of behavioural and drug therapy.

➤ **Behavioural therapy**

➤ Resocialisation and exercise with more walks and excursions that allow the dog to interact with other dogs and individuals from other species.

➤ Establish strong leadership over the dog by practising dominance exercises (see Chapter 1) to improve the owner–dog bond.

It is important to explain to owners that they must be familiar with and meet their dog's behavioural needs, otherwise they should consider rehousing the dog with another family.

➤ **Drug treatment:** the pharmacological groups of choice are benzodiaze-pines (bromazepam, clonazepam, and alprazolam) and nonbenzodiaz-epine anxiolytics belonging to the azapirones group, such as buspirone. SSRIs such as paroxetine can also help. Recommended dosages are:

  ➤ Bromazepam/clonazepam: 0.5–2.0 mg/kg/day in 2–3 doses, orally.
  ➤ Alprazolam: 0.25–2.0 mg/kg/day spread over 2–3 oral doses.
  ➤ Buspirone: 2.5–10.0 mg/animal/day given orally in 2–3 doses.
  ➤ Paroxetine: 0.5–1.0 mg/kg/day in a oral single dose, depending on the size of the dog.

> Whenever a potential owner enquires about the decision to integrate a pet dog into the family, vets must make them understand that dogs have behavioural needs which owners are obliged to meet.

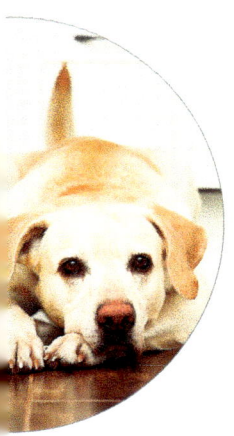

PHOBIAS

A phobia is an amplified fear reaction, a reaction that goes far beyond a normal adaptive response, triggered by an identifiable stimulus.

Fear is a normal adaptive behaviour in dogs, and in basically all species, since it is relatively effective defence mechanism when faced with a potential danger. However, when this fearful reaction develops into an exaggerated response, it transforms from being a beneficial adaptive conduct into a behavioural alteration.

> A phobia is an intense fear response, in fact, the intensity is far greater than that of the actual threat stimulating the reaction.

BEHAVIOURAL DISORDERS IN DOGS

In cases of phobia, dogs are immersed in a state of heighten anxiety that provokes abnormal behaviours: the destruction of objects, inappropriate elimination, excessive vocalisation, attempts to escape, and sometimes aggression towards themselves or others (Figs. 6 and 7).

Pet dogs frequently develop phobias. The most typical stimuli are thunder, storms, gunshots, and fireworks.

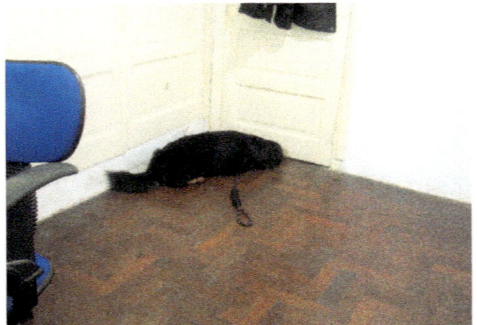

Figure 6. A dog with a phobia displaying an abnormal behaviour by lying next to the room's door.

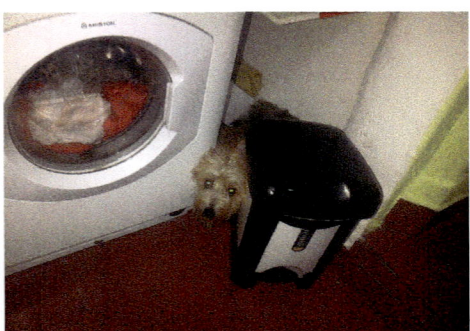

Figure 7. Some dogs with phobias tend to hide.

There are two main types of phobia:
➤ **Ontogenetic phobias:** these start to develop during a dog's socialisation period (when 3–15 weeks old). In this case, there are three different situations that determine the intensity of an individual's reaction to a given stimulus:
  ➤ Situation A: the stimulus occurs regularly and under circumstances that allow for a flight response from the dog. The fear reaction will steadily diminish, and the animal will gradually get used to the given stimulus.
  ➤ Situation B: the stimulus occurs regularly, but the dog cannot exhibit a flight or avoidance behaviour because of the environmental conditions. This complicates the dog's habituation, as it will become sensitised to this stimulus and possibly to other similar stimuli (generalisation process).

➤ Situation C: dogs that were not exposed to the stimulus during their socialisation period. In this case, the animal has not been habituated, so when exposed to the stimulus, it could experience an even more pronounced fear response.

➤ **Reactionary or posttraumatic phobias:** these are acquired after the socialisation period. They can arise at any time in a dog's life and are caused by a traumatic experience. The trigger could be a one-off and generally very violent, shocking event for the dog; on the other hand, it could be a relatively nonviolent but repetitive incident which the dog cannot escape or avoid.

> It is extremely difficult to categorically determine whether a phobia is ontogenetic or posttraumatic.

THE ROLE OF OWNERS IN PHOBIAS

Owner participation is decisive in canine phobias, since they depend on the dog's genetics and living environment, just like all dog behaviours. We can state that an individual's genetic predisposition to exhibit a behavioural response and its environment determine the type and degree of this response.

Owners often unintentionally reinforce their dog's hyperattachment and aggressive behaviour. This means that owners become an aggravating factor in the development of their dog's phobias, when they should really be a fundamental part of the solution.

PATHOGENESIS

Fear is a physiological reaction controlled by adrenaline. However, overstimulation of the adrenergic system and sensitisation cause the dopaminergic system to swing into action and emotional anticipation becomes apparent. This anticipation will cause the phobic behaviour to extend to other situations similar to that of the initial triggering stimulus in a phenomenon called generalisation.

> **Stage 1 (simple phobia):** in this initial phase, the adrenergic reaction is normal and adaptive, although slightly exaggerated. It is called a simple phobia because the dog cannot identify and avoid the triggering stimulus. Externally observable signs are tremors, mydriasis, and anal sac evacuation.

> **Stage 2 (complex phobia):** overstimulation of the adrenergic system and the sensitisation phenomena trigger the dopaminergic system and the emotional anticipation is evident. This anticipation means the phobic behaviour will extend to other situations akin to the initial triggering stimulus in a process known as generalisation. The animal will try to avoid the situation and may develop organic clinical signs including digestive problems (vomiting and diarrhoea), salivation, hypermotility, agitation, hypervigilance, and hypersensitivity, all of which could produce aggressive responses. In this stage, dogs can develop a pathological level of attachment to their owners (hyperattachment).

> **Stage 3:** this situation rarely occurs in practice and can almost be considered a theoretical stage in which the clinical signs from stage 2 are overdimensioned and the animal resigns itself to the fact that it cannot avoid the triggering stimulus. This could be interpreted as a period of rest, but in reality, the dog is in a state of extreme anxiety.

DIAGNOSIS

The diagnosis relies on information collected during the anamnesis, so vets need to ask owners various questions, including:

> The dog's age at onset.
> The frequency of the fearful conduct.
> Whether the dog displays aggression or hyperattachment.
> Whether the dog exhibits any external signs during the phobic behaviour.
> Whether the dog has suffered any traumatic events at some point in its lifetime.

The direct observation of the patient's behaviour is also important, even though the dog may not be expressing the phobia during the consultation.

Vets must also rule out any underlying clinical diseases that could cause the behavioural disorder.

- Sociopathies
- Behavioural alterations associated with thyroid disorders
- Hyperattachment to the owner due to other causes

PROGNOSIS

The prognosis varies greatly depending on the length of time since the phobia established itself, the patient's capacity to cope with intense stimuli during treatment, and the owner's capacity and willingness to collaborate in the treatment.

> If the dog has only been exhibiting the phobia for a short period and appears emotionally stable when exposed to the triggering stimulus, and if the owner seems willing to engage in their dog's treatment, then the prognosis is generally good.

TREATMENT

Both behavioural and drug therapy should be used jointly and in a complementary manner.

- **Behavioural therapy:** this is based on the use of two behaviour modification techniques:
  - Systematic desensitisation: this method consists of gradually exposing the dog to the stimulus that provokes its phobic reaction, throughout which the owner should completely ignore the dog's response. It is a very tiresome technique, so owners must be willing and able to learn it and put it into practice. It is commonly applied in the case of animals with a phobia triggered by auditory stimuli.
  - Counterconditioning: this is used together with desensitisation and entails rewarding the dog every time it does not exhibit fear when confronted with the triggering stimulus, thus reinforcing its favourable emotional state. It is essential that owners avoid rewarding the dog's phobic states, so they must be very alert to their pet's reactions and bodily postures. Counterconditioning requires a lot of time and effort; as such, owners must be very willing and engaged.

> **Drug treatment:** phobias can only be corrected through the use of behaviour modification techniques and by altering the dog's environment, but pharmacological treatment is a very important aid to behavioural therapy.

In the simple phobia stage, the aim of drug therapy is to inhibit the internal mechanisms that trigger the fear response using beta-blockers:
> Propranolol: 0.5 mg/kg, every 8 hours, orally. Pay special attention for signs of bradycardia.

The dopaminergic system influences the generalisation of phobias that occurs in stage 2, so the use of neuroleptics is indicated:
> Selegiline: 0.5 mg/kg/day, split over two oral doses.

In the final stage, when inhibition develops, tricyclic antidepressants or SSRIs are recommended:
> Clomipramine: 1–3 mg/kg/day given orally in 2 doses.
> Paroxetine: 0.5–1.0 mg/kg/day in a oral single dose.

Although phenothiazines are routinely used in veterinary medicine, they should be avoided for phobias, since at effective doses they inhibit learning and, therefore, the ability to habituate patients to triggering stimuli.

Another option is the administration of benzodiazepine anxiolytics, mainly those with an antiphobic action:
> Clonazepam: 0.5–2.0 mg/kg/day in two doses taken orally.
> Alprazolam: 0.25–2.0 mg/kg/day in 2–3 oral doses.

Azapirone derivative anxiolytics can also treat phobias:
> Buspirone: 2.5–10.0 mg/animal/day given in two oral doses.

> Always try to administer the lowest effective dose of the drug for each patient, as such the dosage should be adjusted as the treatment advances.

AGORAPHOBIA AND SOCIAL PHOBIA

Dogs that display a fear of people (Fig. 8), other animals, and public spaces in general have agoraphobia or social phobia. They are only in a nonphobic state when in their own home. Some may even exhibit phobic behaviour when a stranger visits the home (Fig. 9).

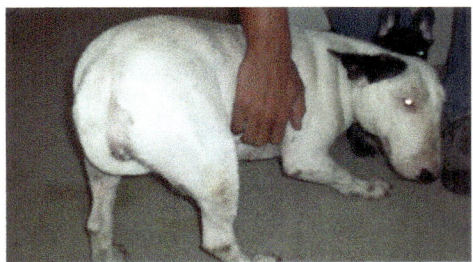

Figure 8. A dog displaying a fearful posture (tail between the legs) when touched.

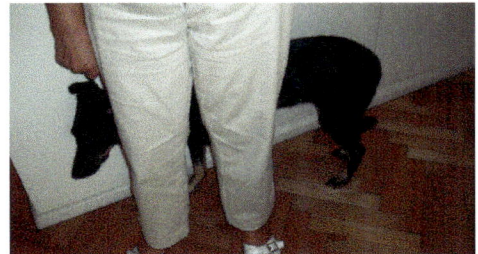

Figure 9. This dog is trying to protect itself behind its owner following the arrival of a visitor.

DIAGNOSIS

The diagnosis is based on data collected in the anamnesis and by direct observation during consultation. It is important to rule out any medical conditions that could be the origin of the behavioural disorder.

TREATMENT

Treatment is founded on systematic desensitisation and gradually exposing the patient to the stimuli that trigger the behavioural alteration. Punishment is strictly and specifically contraindicated when treating agoraphobia or social phobia.

Recommended antiphobic anxiolytics are the benzodiazepines:
➤ Clonazepam: 0.5–2.0 mg/kg/day in 2-3 doses taken orally.
➤ Alprazolam: 0.25–2.0 mg/kg/day spread over 2–3 oral doses.

PHOBIA OF LOUD NOISES OR STORMS

This problem is generally encountered in dogs aged 2–3 years, both in males and females, and there is not enough evidence to determine whether the incidence differs between breeds.

DIAGNOSIS

The diagnosis relies on information from the anamnesis, as well as observation of the dog and its interaction with its owner during consultation.

TREATMENT

Treatment revolves around systematic desensitisation and punishment is contraindicated. In practice, the objective is to habituate the animal to the stimulus (loud bangs, storms, strong winds, etc.) so it remains calm throughout the event.

Antiphobic anxiolytics are generally used to complement behavioural therapy:
➤ Clonazepam: 0.5–2.0 mg/kg/day in 2–3 oral doses.
➤ Alprazolam: 0.25–2.0 mg/animal/day in 2–3 oral doses.

Tranquillisers such as acetylpromazine should be used with precaution due to their side effects, which include a diminished learning capacity.

COMPULSIVE DISORDERS

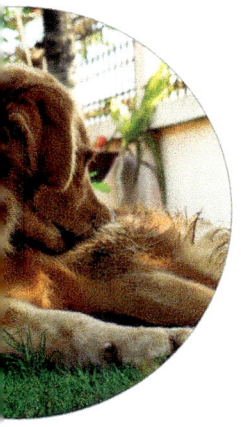

A compulsive behaviour, or stereotypy, is a persistent, repetitive action with no apparent purpose. This definition is not strictly accurate, as stereotypies have different degrees of variation. Some are repetitive acts (e.g. animals that remain stationary for a certain amount of time) and others, although repetitive, have a clear aim (scratching or grooming).

> Patients feel an uncontrollable impulse to act out stereotypies even though they do not derive any pleasure from them. They are not just an exaggeration of a normal behaviour, rather a pathological deviation of a specific conduct (grooming, vocalisation, locomotion, etc.).

It is a very common behavioural disorder in pet dogs and originates from specific neuropathological changes caused by variations in brain biochemistry.

The best-known stereotyped behaviours in dogs are tail chasing and mutilation (Fig. 10), walking in circles, incessant leg licking resulting in dermatological lesions (Fig. 11), and constant flank sucking (Fig. 12).

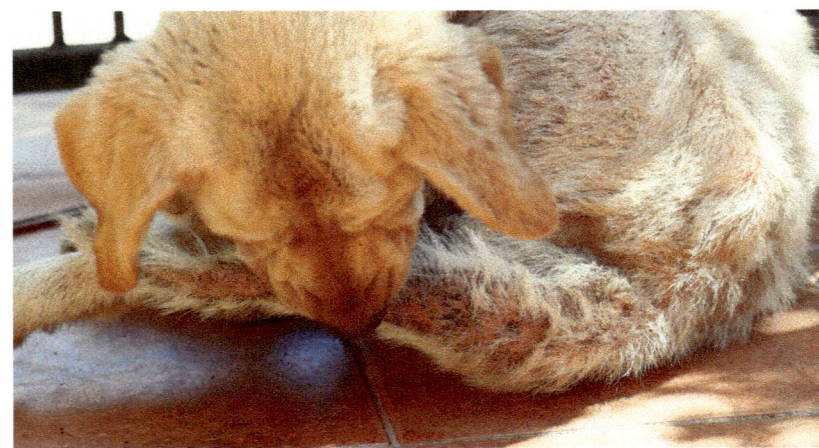

Figure 10.
Some dogs bite and mutilate their tail.

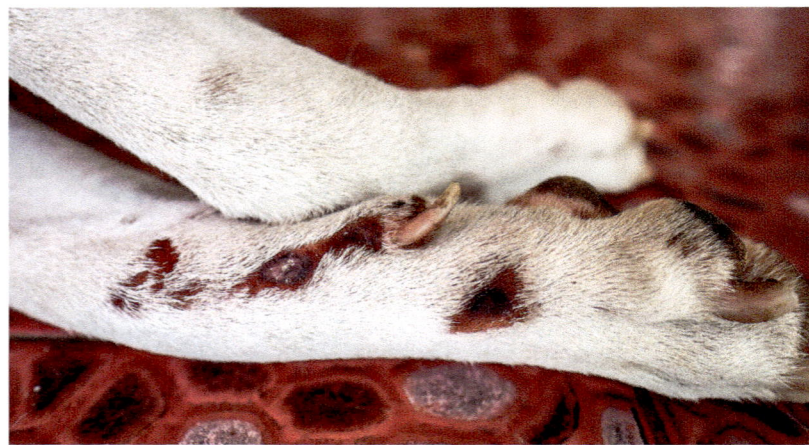

Figure 11.
Chronic leg licking can produce dermatological lesions.

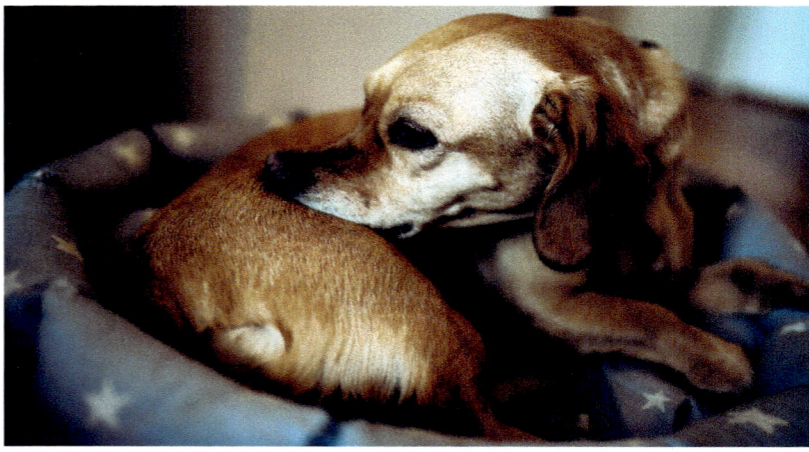

Figure 12.
Constant flank sucking is another stereotyped behaviour.

TYPES OF STEREOTYPIES IN DOGS

The various compulsive disorders observed in dogs are categorised according to the normal motor patterns from which they deviate:

- ➤ Grooming disorders: compulsive licking, hair chewing, acral granulomas, etc.
- ➤ Hallucinations: chattering teeth, hunting nonexistent prey, staring into space, etc.
- ➤ Eating disorders: polydipsia, polyphagia, pica (ingesting nonfood items), etc.
- ➤ Locomotion disorders: sudden body movements, running and jumping, remaining stationary, walking in circles, etc.
- ➤ Vocalisation: constant barking or whining, etc.
- ➤ Neurosis: self-mutilation with or without vocalisation, sudden aggression towards people or other animals, etc.

PATHOGENESIS

Four important genes have been isolated in people with obsessive–compulsive disorder and their mutations may be responsible for altered levels of serotonin, a neurotransmitter associated with the development of various conditions such as anxiety, stress, certain phobias, and depression. One of these genes is HTR2A, which codes for a serotonin receptor.

Scientific studies in dogs have also connected compulsive canine behaviour to specific genes. For example, a study published in Molecular Psychiatry demonstrated that Dobermanns that licked their flanks compulsively shared a gene.

Furthermore, a canine chromosome 7 locus was discovered to contain the gene CDH2 (cadherin-2, type 0, N-cadherin), a genetic variation observed in dogs that lick themselves compulsively. The CDH2 gene codes for cadherin, a protein involved in cell alignment, adhesion, and communication.

Recent calculations suggest that up to 8 % of dogs in the USA (5–6 million animals) exhibit compulsive behaviours such as fence running, pacing across small spaces, circling, tail chasing, biting imaginary flies, licking, biting, barking, and staring into space. Researchers have also found a higher incidence of compulsive disorders among males compared to females (in a 3:1 ratio), while this ratio is the opposite in cats.

Ultimately, as is the case with most behavioural alterations, the aetiology and pathogenesis of this disorder are both genetic and environmental, so they can be classified as either pathophysiological conditions (inherited or acquired) or experiential alterations (traumatic or negative experiences at some time in the dog's life).

In fact a lack of adequate socialisation during the crucial period of 3–15 weeks of age can predispose dogs to exhibit stereotyped behaviours as adults, even though they live in a suitable environment. Regardless of the origin, most dogs with a compulsive disorder also suffer from very high levels of generalised anxiety.

DIAGNOSIS

A diagnosis can be reached by observing the patient's behaviour and from information collected during the anamnesis.

The likelihood of carrying out genetic studies that would conclusively provide an accurate diagnosis is rather improbable in veterinary medicine, at least for the time being.

It is very important to rule out clinical diseases as an underlying cause of the compulsive disorder.

> The prognosis ranges from reserved to severe depending on whether the compulsive disorder is genetic, acquired, or a combination thereof.

TREATMENT

The cause of the conflict needs to be identified and withdrawn, and the animal should never be punished or physically prevented from acting out the stereotypy.

The treatment of compulsive disorders requires the use of some specific behaviour modification techniques in combination with drug therapy, as it is practically impossible to resolve the problem without it.

- ➤ **Behavioural therapy:** this should consist of:
  - ➤ Avoiding all punishment.
  - ➤ Curbing the behaviour by indirectly diverting the dog's attention, but without the dog associating its compulsive behaviour with attention from its owner.
  - ➤ Environmental enrichment. Owners must understand that their dog's behavioural needs are just as important as its physical needs and it must be allowed to exhibit and execute the normal behaviours expected of its species.

- ➤ **Drug treatment:** the drugs of choice are SSRIs and serotonin modulators. Anticonvulsants, sedatives, and tranquilizers are not usually effective in the treatment of stereotyped conducts.

  Given that most cases of compulsive behaviour are accompanied by a high level of anxiety, anxiolytics are also usually coadministered.

  Several types of drug can be used, but if the chosen drug does not produce the desired results, it should be changed for another one:
  - ➤ Buspirone: 2.5–10.0 mg/animal/day given in two oral doses.
  - ➤ Paroxetine: 0.5–1.0 mg/kg/day in a oral single dose.
  - ➤ Clomipramine: 1–3 mg/kg/day in a oral single dose.
  - ➤ Bromazepam: 0.5–2.0 mg/kg/day in 2–3 oral doses.
  - ➤ Alprazolam: 0.25–2.0 mg/kg/day in 2–3 oral doses.

COMPULSIVE DISORDERS ASSOCIATED WITH EATING BEHAVIOUR

There are several compulsive conducts related to eating habits, and although they are essentially the same as other behavioural disorders with respect to their diagnosis, prognosis, and treatment, vets and owners should be aware of their implications.

➤ **Pica:** this is when dogs eat nonfood substances such as rags, plastic, or wooden objects, and so on.

➤ **Stone chewing:** compulsively chewing on stones, dogs may even wear their teeth down so much that they are notably smoother.

➤ **Polydipsia/polyphagia:** drinking water and eating compulsively. This can lead to obesity, which is another very common anxiety-related disorder.

COMPULSIVE DISORDERS ASSOCIATED WITH LOCOMOTION

➤ **Excessive ambulation:** compulsively walking in circles or a figure-of-eight. It is frequently observed in German and Belgian Shepherds. Dogs will only stop this behaviour when fatigued and as soon as they regain some energy, they will start ambulating again. It is also common among dogs that live in cages or kennels.

➤ **Scratching the ground:** compulsively scratching the floor with their paws and nails, regardless of what the ground is made of (Fig. 13).

➤ **Tail chasing:** patients that walk in circles, stop and try to bite their tail. After a few attempts, they will start circling again. This is often observed along with excessive ambulation.

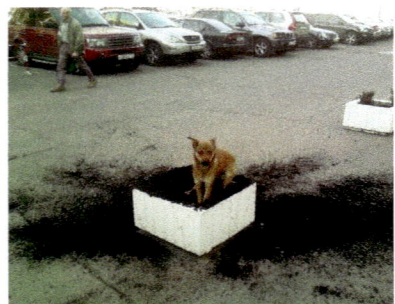

Figure 13. A dog compulsively scratching the ground, without regard to the type of surface or its location.

COMPULSIVE DISORDERS ASSOCIATED WITH VOCALISATION

➤ **Incessant barking/howling:** barking or howling compulsively and without any recognisable occurrence that triggers the behaviour.
➤ **Barking at food bowl:** barking compulsively at the dog's food bowl. Sometimes they do it for a few minutes and then eat; on other occasions, they bark constantly and repetitively even though the bowl is empty.

VARIOUS NEUROSES

➤ **Acral granulomas due to excessive licking:** in this case dogs lick their legs continually and repetitively, which thickens the epidermis and provokes a granuloma. They usually do this while lying down, so the acral granulomas are almost always located on the carpi and tarsi, as they are easily accessed from a lying position (Fig. 14).

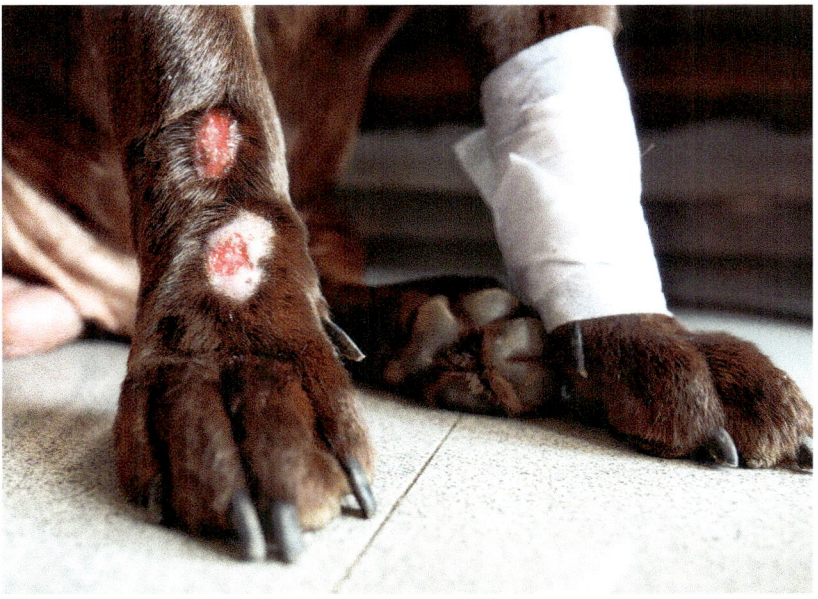

Figure 14. Acral granuloma on the carpus.

> **Flank sucking:** dogs start by licking their flanks and end up sucking on it. This often causes local dermatitis and subsequently a bacterial infection.

> **Chasing nonexistent flies:** constantly trying to trap imaginary flies. Retinal diseases must be ruled out via an eye fundus examination before the problem can be diagnosed as a compulsive behavioural disorder.

> **Nail biting (onychophagy):** compulsively biting nails until bloody and painful, but even then, the dog will continue to exhibit the conduct.

> **Unpredictable aggression:** animals that attack savagely and for no apparent reason. In the past, this behavioural alteration was associated with anxiety, but nowadays it is linked to subclinical motor epilepsy. Therefore, epilepsy should be investigated as an underlying cause, in which case an electroencephalogram would reveal an epileptogenic focus that does not reach the necessary threshold to trigger convulsions.

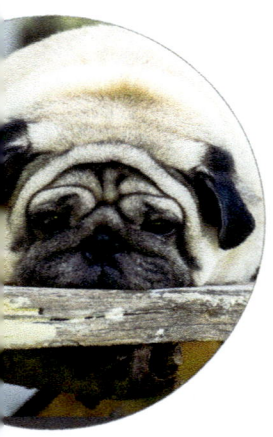

OTHER BEHAVIOURAL DISORDERS ASSOCIATED WITH ANXIETY

COPROPHAGY

Coprophagy is the ingestion of faeces, both its own and that of other dogs, with independence of sex, age, or breed.

> Coprophagy in puppies can be considered normal, but in adults it corresponds to an anxiety-related behavioural disorder.

Vets should determine whether the animal realises the behaviour in front of its owner, in order to differentiate it from a call for social attention. They must also pay special attention to the dog–owner relationship to ascertain the degree of attachment and bonding between them.

Any clinical conditions related to the digestive process should be ruled out. The prognosis is good, but it should be cautious.

Treatment is based on the use of anxiolytics and enriching the dog's environment. More physical activity and keeping the dog entertained also help a great deal. Where possible, the dog's access to faeces should be restricted.

OBESITY

Obesity has traditionally been considered a clinical problem with origins in glandular or hormonal disorders, metabolic alterations, a genetic predisposition, and so on. Nowadays, an ever-increasing number of medical professionals agree that it can also be due to a behavioural disorder associated with anxiety.

Certain breeds and female dogs are more predisposed to develop anxiety-related obesity, as they show a higher incidence than other populations. Another factor that affects obesity in dogs is castration, particularly in the case of females.

DIAGNOSIS

Diagnosis revolves around information from the anamnesis and direct observation of the owner–dog relationship. In general, there are signs of the dog's excessive attachment to its owners, who are usually overly protective (Fig. 15). The presence of any underlying diseases must be ruled out.

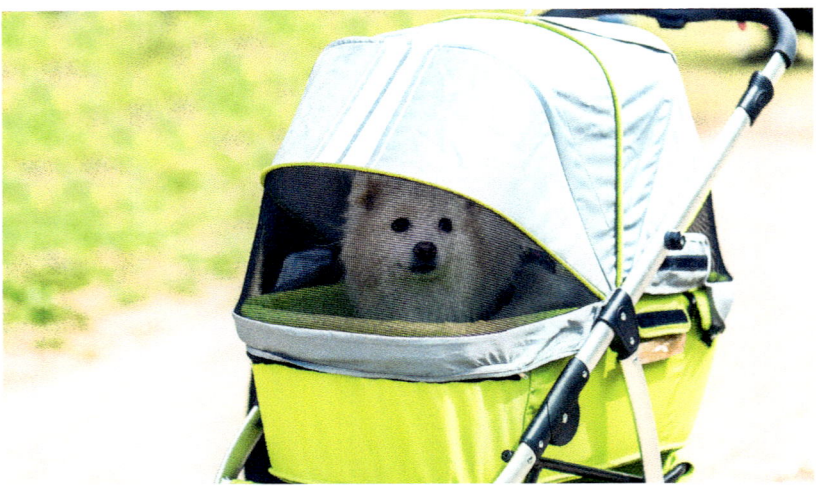

Figure 15. Some owners overindulge their dogs, and this prevents them from exhibiting normal behavioural patterns inherent to their species.

PROGNOSIS

While the prognosis should be positive, it primarily depends on the owners, because even though the behavioural therapy is simple enough, many are still unable to put it into practice.

TREATMENT

Treatment is based on trying to reduce the dog's food intake. This can be achieved by gradually reducing the amount of food given to the animal each day or by completely fasting for a few days. Both methods have their advocates and opponents, but either way, a dog's eating habits can definitely be changed through the gradual reduction of its daily calorie intake.

More daily physical activity (long walks) and a change in owner handling are undoubtedly essential factors in achieving therapeutic success.

> It is vital that owners understand the risk that obesity represents to their dog's health.

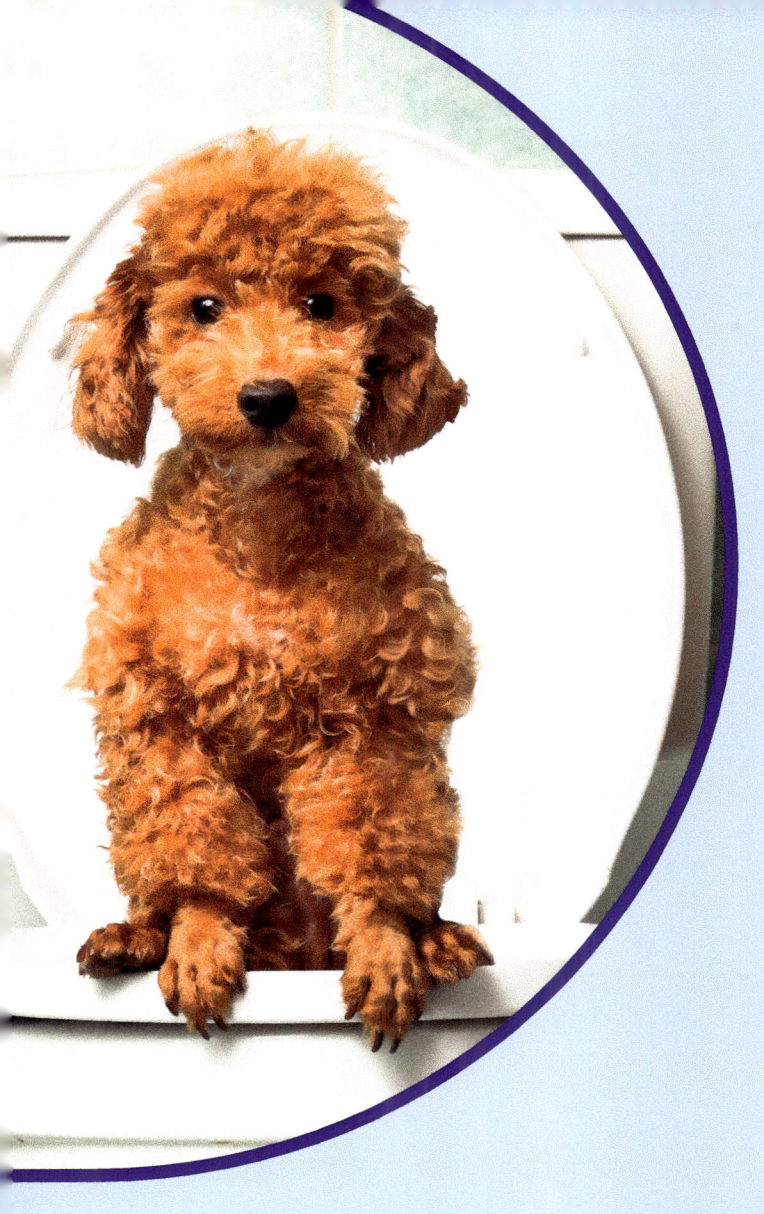

DISORDERS ASSOCIATED WITH ELIMINATION BEHAVIOUR

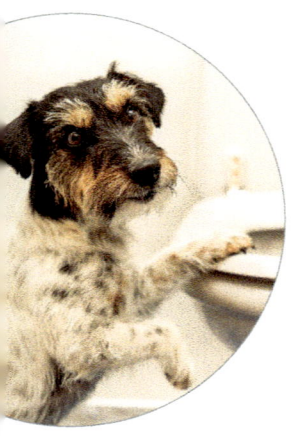

INTRODUCTION

In daily veterinary practice, a high percentage of ethology consultations for pet dogs are concerned with elimination behaviour problems. This is mainly because owners find this type of abnormal behaviour particularly disagreeable. As occurs with other conducts, elimination behaviour is influenced by both genetic and environmental factors.

Elimination behaviour refers to both urination and defaecation and it merges with a dog's communicative and social behaviour. This means, that for basically didactic purposes, it is hard to group them together under a single type of behaviour. Urination and defaecation can also occur in contexts related to other behavioural patterns and may often be concomitant with elevated levels of anxiety, for example in the case of separation anxiety, fear, or phobias.

During the neonatal period (first 2 weeks of life), a puppy's elimination behaviour is totally involuntary, as the mother has to lick her offspring's perineal area to induce the reflex that voids their physiological waste, which the female will ingest to complete the process. Little by little, while in their third week, the puppies will start to evacuate voluntarily and increasingly further away from the nest until eventually, at the age of about 9 weeks, they do it in specific locations.

Urinary elimination behaviour in pet dogs, and the corresponding posture, differs between adult males and females (sexual dimorphism) and depends on the organising effects of sex hormones during the first few months of life. In fact, these differences are evident before puppies reach puberty, as prepubescent males urinate stood on all fours with their body leaning forwards in a position similar to females. Obviously, after puberty the disparities are much more apparent. Postpubescent female dogs continue to lower their hindquarters when urinating (Fig. 1), while males raise one of their back legs (Fig. 2), although a small proportion of individuals may take up intermediate postures. Sex hormones increase urinary frequency; in females, chiefly during oestrus to increase the excretion of hormones that attract males; and in males, the periodicity increases for territorial marking purposes, which is also related to social hierarchy since the rate is higher among dominant dogs. However, there is no sexual dimorphism with respect to defaecation posture.

Urination, besides eliminating waste, fulfils a communication function based on the canine olfactory system, in which urine and other bodily fluids are the source of chemical stimuli. It is generally related to territorial marking, but this is not its only function.

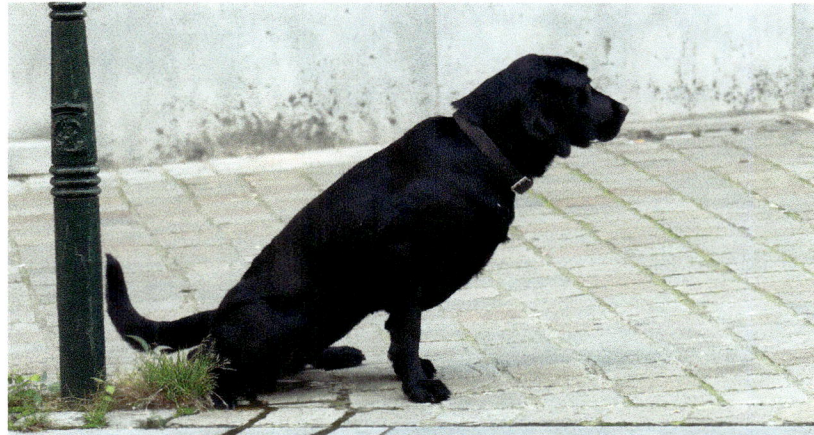

Figure 1. Females lower their hindquarters when urinating.

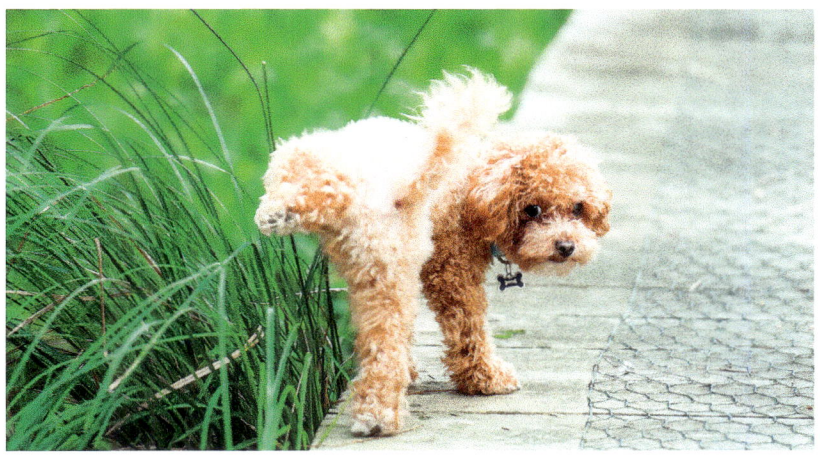

Figure 2. Male dogs cock one of their back legs during urination.

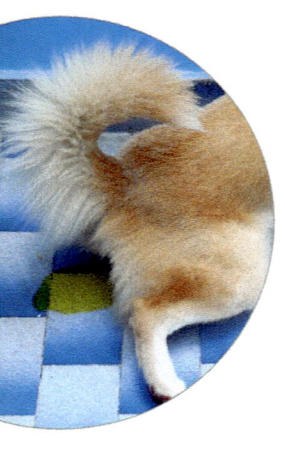

ELIMINATION IN INAPPROPRIATE LOCATIONS

When assessing this behaviour, the first thing to consider is the patient's age, as a puppy's main aim is to simply discard waste, whereas in adults it may be associated with communication between peers. Notwithstanding, veterinary surgeons should also assess the possibility of a fear response, anxiety, or excitement in both adults and puppies.

DIAGNOSIS

The diagnosis is made according to information collected during the anamnesis.

Rule out any medical conditions that course with pollakiuria, incontinence, or episodes of diarrhoea, and any which affect locomotion or cause pain when in the urination or defaecation posture (arthritis, disc diseases, etc.).

After ruling out a clinical cause, the diagnosis should focus on differentiating between the possible scenarios:

➤ Fear response: some dogs cannot control their sphincters in the presence of a stimulus that triggers fear or panic such as a violent owner, thunder, storms, or individuals that frighten them.

➤ Separation anxiety: dogs can enter into a state of extreme anxiety when left alone which they channel by urinating or defaecating wherever they find themselves at that moment rather than in their usual locations.

➤ Incorrect training: dogs that have been raised incorrectly or in small spaces (patios, cages, etc.) may eliminate inappropriately and continue with this behavioural pattern even after being relocated, unless they are suitably retrained.

> Regardless of the initial cause, the prognosis is good because in most cases appropriate retraining yields successful outcomes.

TREATMENT

Treatment is mainly based on behavioural therapy and does not involve any drugs. Evidently, it will depend on the cause of the problem, but a possible treatment plan for consideration is to:

➤ Treat or manage the likely underlying medical problems.

➤ Retrain the dog by positively reinforcing elimination in correct locations.

➤ Increase the amount of outdoor physical activity.

➤ Condition the dog to avoid the behaviour by completely removing the odour from the location of undesired elimination (Fig. 3), by blocking the dog's access to the location, and so on.

> If possible, place the dog's food and water bowls in the inappropriate location where it is eliminating.

Never overly or physically punish the animal, although owners can reprimand them if they catch them in the act.

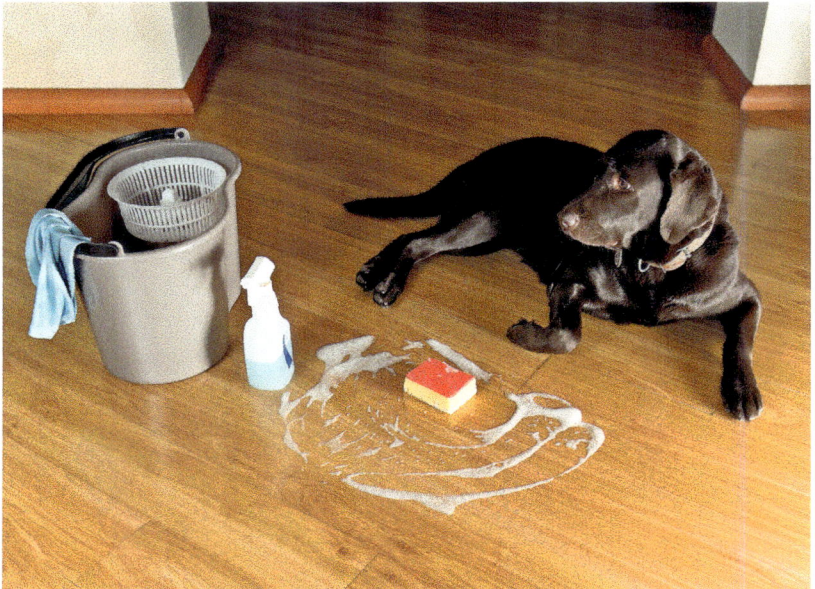

Figure 3. It is essential to thoroughly clean the area where the dog eliminates to prevent odours.

BEHAVIOURAL DISORDERS IN DOGS

ELIMINATION RETRAINING

Success in elimination retraining depends on the owner's constant supervision, patience, and persistence, both with respect to constraining eliminations in undesired locations and reinforcing those in the correct situations.

Dogs should be fed a low-residue diet, preferably just once a day, during the retraining process.

Whenever the dog eliminates in the wrong place while the owner is present, they should scold the animal without being aggressive or violent, but they should be firm and immediately take it to an appropriate location for elimination (Fig. 4). It helps to place the dog's food and water bowls in the area of inappropriate eliminations.

In extreme and refractory cases, owners can use an appropriately sized transport cage whenever they have to leave their pet unattended or uncontrolled. They can also use small, enclosed areas around the home (patio, kitchen, laundry room, etc.).

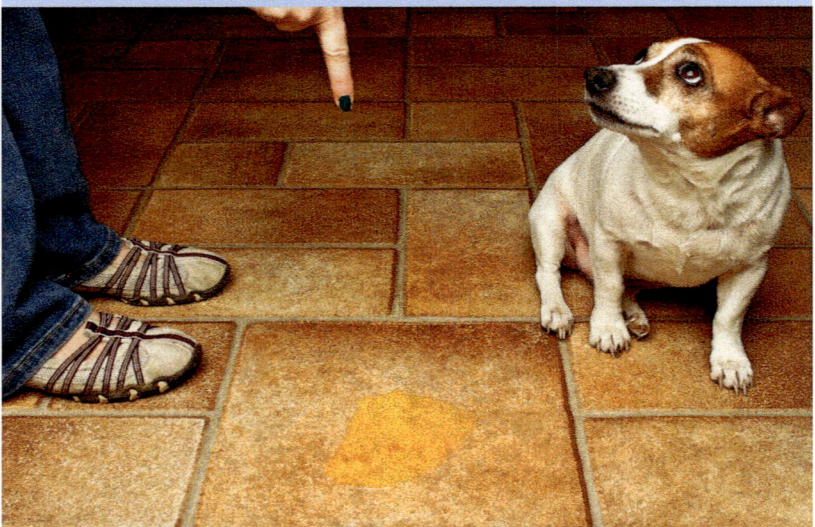

Figure 4. Owners should reprimand adult dogs, without being aggressive or violent, when they eliminate in an appropriate location.

PREVENTION

The best means of preventing this behavioural disorder is, without a doubt, appropriate training. There are two different situations: training a puppy and retraining an adult dog in order to treat a patient that already presents the problem.

As such, owners should pay attention to when their puppy is about to eliminate in an undesired location, pick it up and take it to a correctly prepared area (with absorbent material on the floor) while praising it with adulation (Fig. 5), as rewarding it with food is ill-advised. When the puppy is left alone, it should be confined to the space that contains the area prepared for its eliminations. This technique should be used until the puppy starts to go out for walks in the street. It should be lavished with praise whenever it eliminates during a walk. Owners must never use a correction technique that prompts a fear response in the puppy.

There is a possibility that the longer the process of conditioning the animal to eliminate in the prepared indoor area continues, then the longer it takes to condition it to eliminate outside during walks; therefore, it is important to introduce the puppy to walks as soon as possible. To this end, some of the vaccinations currently available provide correct immunisation against the most prevalent viral diseases before puppies reach the end of the socialisation period, which spans from the age of 3 to 12–15 weeks.

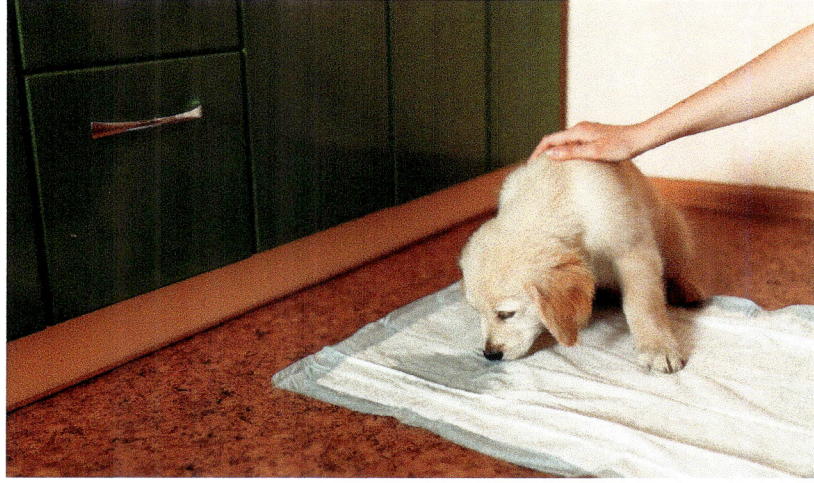

Figure 5. Never forget to congratulate the puppy when it eliminates in the location prepared for this purpose.

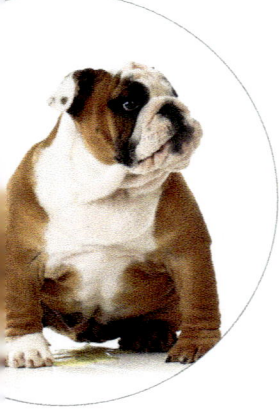

MARKING

Marking is an important form of communication between domestic dogs, as it involves more than just excretory organs and the olfactory system. The central nervous system is responsible for receiving, regulating, and determining the eventual behavioural response to marking.

> Both hormones and neurotransmitters play an important role in this means of communication.

DIAGNOSIS

When dealing with a patient with an elimination behaviour disorder, the first step is to determine whether the problem relates to inappropriate elimination or marking, which is easily established through the anamnesis.

Generally speaking, in the case of elimination behaviour, dogs excrete a lot of urine in a single location, whereas marking behaviour involves small amounts at various sites. Although it is not as obvious as in cats, the two postures also tend to differ, especially in the case of urination, but it can be so subtle that owners rarely notice it.

An important point to ascertain during the anamnesis is whether or not the dog has been castrated, particularly if it is a male, as males manifest this behaviour more than females. The dog's age is another important factor, given that marking is mainly carried out by young adults.

During the anamnesis, owners often mention that their dog generally marks after becoming frustrated; for instance, after barking through the window at a dog in the street or when it is physically separated from a certain member of the household. Another common situation reported by owners is dogs that urinate on the owner's favourite sofa or armchair (Fig. 6).

> Pay attention to other behaviours unrelated to elimination that could reveal information about the social relationship between the dog and its owners.

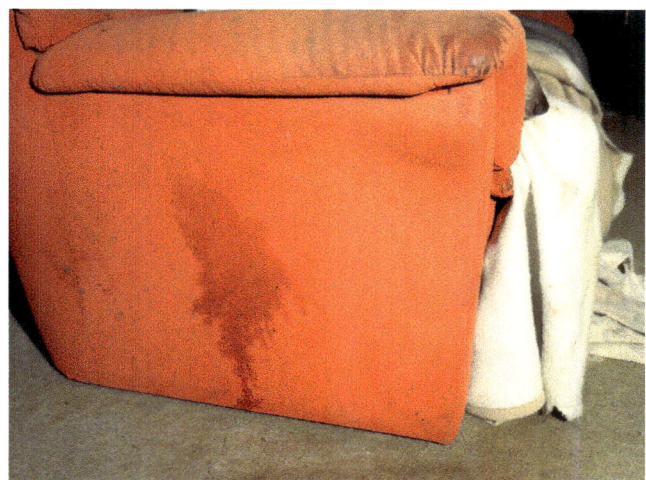

Figure 6. Urine marks on a sofa from a male dog.

Behavioural alterations related to marking in pet dogs are strongly linked to, and often accompanied by, other disorders related to the patient's aggressive and social behaviours.

The diagnosis is fairly straightforward and is made according to data collected in the anamnesis, while always ruling out any associated underlying clinical diseases.

> The prognosis is relatively good, but it will depend on the owner's willingness, patience, and commitment to practising the behavioural therapy.

BEHAVIOURAL DISORDERS IN DOGS

TREATMENT

- **Surgical treatment:** surgical castration is indicated for intact males and has a high success rate, since it reduces marking behaviour in 50 % of cases. It is also recommended for intact females, although the success rate is lower.
- **Behavioural therapy:** this involves conditioning the dog in order to inhibit the behaviour. Remote punishment devices are helpful when dogs cannot be supervised. The remote punishment should be an aversive stimulus for the dog, with enough intensity to deter its behaviour but without inducing fear and without the dog associating it with its owner's presence. Some electronic devices are now available that release a spray when the dog breaks a light beam.

PREVENTION

Marking is more closely related to agonistic behaviour than any other type of conduct, so it is crucial that owners exert leadership over their dog to avoid competition for the hierarchical position. Confrontations with the dog can range from defiance (through territorial marking around the home) to aggression towards a family member.

FAECAL MARKING

Marking with faeces is very rare among pet dogs that live inside a home. In faecal marking, after defaecating the dog will scratch the ground energetically using its hindlimbs to disperse the odour impregnated in the faeces. This odour is secreted from the perianal glands located within the anal sacs. Dominant and very self-confident dogs scratch the floor more vigorously after defaecating.

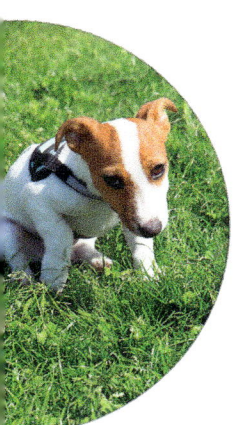

SUBMISSIVE URINATION

Submissive urination is related to a dog's social rank. Although it can be observed in dogs of any age, it is much more frequent in puppies and young females.

The triggering stimulus is normally a dominant adult dog and sometimes an excessively strict owner.

When in the presence of the intimidating individual, the patient will adopt a submissive posture and involuntarily start to urinate (it will roll onto its back while releasing streams of urine) (Fig. 7).

This problem usually resolves itself during the dog's development, as it progressively gains self-confidence, and therefore the cases that are brought to the clinic tend to be persistent and harder to remedy.

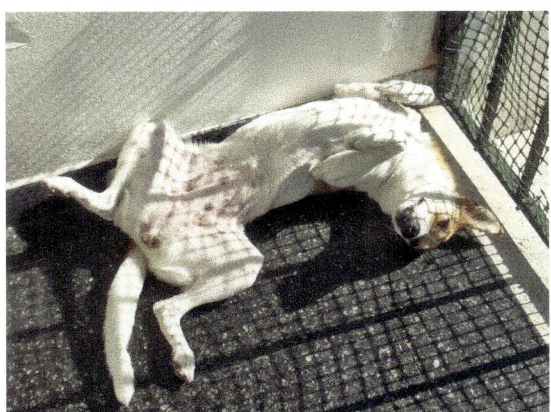

Figure 7. A young female dog in a submissive position.

DIAGNOSIS

Diagnosis relies on information collected during the anamnesis and through direct observation of the patient's behaviour. Any nonbehavioural causes must be ruled out. The prognosis is good in most cases.

TREATMENT

Treatment focuses on behaviour modification techniques:

- ➤ **Counterconditioning:** this comprises teaching dogs to practise a behaviour that is incompatible with the submissive state and urination. For example, owners can order their dog to execute a simple command such as sitting and award it with a toy when it complies. Then, when in the presence of an intimidating individual, the owner should distract the dog with the same toy. This behaviour can be reinforced through modelling: at first, the dog should complete the learnt behaviour and be rewarded, then it should only be rewarded if it maintains a sitting position when greeted by the intimidating individual, and finally, instead of giving it the toy when it continues to sit, the owner should just lightly congratulate and stroke their dog.
- ➤ **Systematic desensitisation:** this technique is based on increasingly exposing the dog in a gradual and controlled manner to the stimulus that triggers the submissive urination behaviour. It should be applied in combination with counterconditioning techniques.

> Physical punishment is strictly contraindicated.

PREVENTION

Prevention consists of correct, nonintimidating handling of puppies. Excessively submissive dogs require a lot of patience from their owners and help building their confidence. Obedience training based on positive reinforcement is an excellent means of achieving this goal.

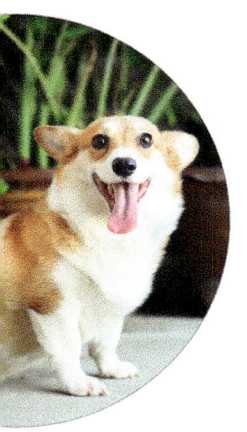

EXCITEMENT URINATION

Excitement urination is similar to submissive urination, but dogs do not adopt submissive behaviours or postures as there is no fear-based component. Rather it is excessive excitement that causes dogs to urinate profusely and involuntarily.

DIAGNOSIS

This problem can be diagnosed through the anamnesis and direct observation of the dog's behaviour.

> Excitement urination normally occurs in the presence of someone with whom the dog has a strong emotional bond.

TREATMENT

➤ **Behavioural therapy:** treatment involves counterconditioning, distraction techniques, and obedience training, as well as more outdoor physical activity. Too many or inappropriate rewards may further excite the patient, so they are not indicated during this type of treatment.

➤ **Drug treatment:** medications are used as an aid to behavioural therapy. The tricyclic antidepressant imipramine at an oral dosage of 1–3 mg/kg every 12 or 24 hours helps increase sphincter muscle tone. It is usually used in the most uncontrollable cases or those refractory to behavioural therapy.

PREVENTION

The prevention of excitement urination involves an assessment of each puppy's personality so that it may be trained accordingly. It is important to avoid greeting puppies with too much enthusiasm if they tend to be very nervous in certain situations.

URINARY INCONTINENCE

Urinary incontinence is due to medical causes, so a clinical examination is necessary to detect any disorders (physiological anomalies, bacterial infections, neurovegetative disorders, tumours, diabetes insipidus, etc.).

Castrated dogs, mainly females due to a lack of oestrogens, and elderly dogs, due to cognitive dysfunction, can suffer from urinary incontinence.

Treatment comprises the use of psychoactive and hormonal medications. The most commonly used drugs are:

➤ Imipramine: 1–3 mg/kg every 12 or 24 hours, orally.

➤ Oestrogens/testosterone: depending on each case and at dosages used in clinical practice.

➤ Monoamine oxidase B inhibitors (MAO-B inhibitors): oral selegiline is used at a dosage of 0.5 mg/kg twice/day in elderly dogs with cognitive dysfunction.

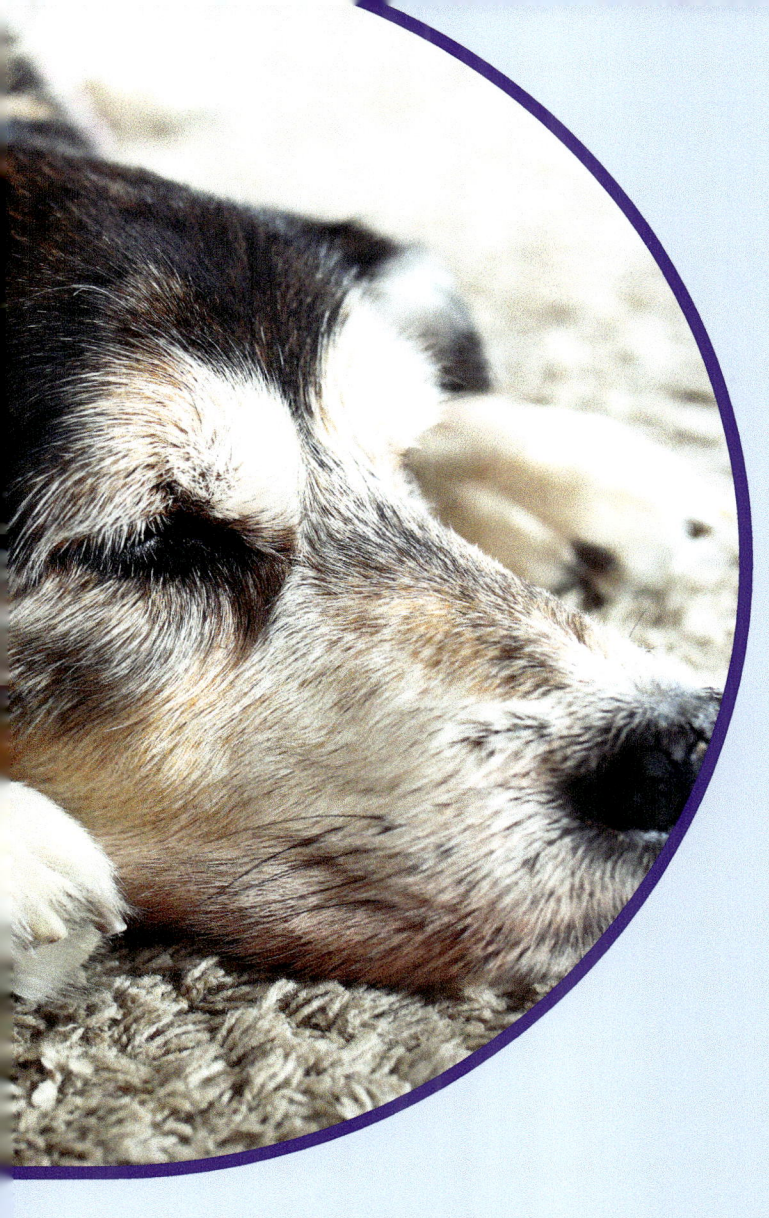

DISORDERS ASSOCIATED WITH COGNITIVE DECLINE

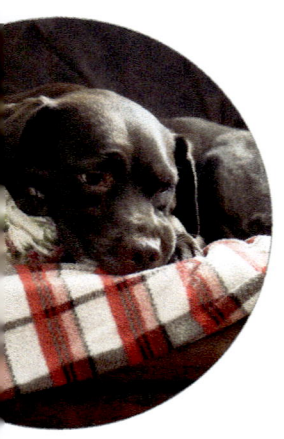

INTRODUCTION

Older dogs, aged between 9 and 11 years, depending on their breed, are not just adult dogs but instead they should be considered geriatric patients.

Domestic animals go through significant changes in old age compared to adulthood. What is more, from an ethological perspective and in contrast to other veterinary specialities, there is a further factor besides the organic changes that affect ageing dogs – owners find it hard to appreciate that their dog's abnormal behaviour is due to its advancing years and therefore they need to learn new forms of interacting with their pet.

As dogs enter into old age, they suffer neurochemical and vascular changes in the brain which can produce cognitive alterations that consequently cause the animal to exhibit abnormal behaviours or which differ from those displayed when it was an adult.

DEGENERATIVE CHANGES IN OLD AGE

The degenerative changes that affect the various organ systems during a dog's senile stage also bear a strong influence on behavioural disorders. Some examples include:

► Osteoarticular disorders (arthritis, spondylosis, etc.): these cause pain and contribute to the chances of an aggressive response when disturbed.
► Urogenital problems (cystitis, prostatomegaly, kidney failure, etc.): can make the dog abandon the appropriate elimination habits it learnt in the past.
► Liver diseases: these can induce a state of intoxication, which in turn contributes to neurological disorders and their associated behavioural alterations.

There are many more, as any organic alteration can affect a dog's behaviour.

It has been shown that dementia in dogs is accompanied by the same changes in neurotransmitters that occur in humans with Alzheimer's disease and senile dementia. Therefore, pets can be treated, but not cured, with medications similar to those used in human medicine (nicergoline, selegiline, etc.).

> The main behavioural disorders in senile dogs are aggression, inappropriate elimination, anxiety, and increased irritability.

Furthermore, elderly animals suffer a decline in their sensory capacities (mainly visual and auditory), so they experience insecurity, stress, and anxiety when faced with everyday situations. They may also present an altered sleep–wake cycle, waking up and becoming active during the night, while sleeping too much during the day (Fig. 1).

It is very difficult to clearly differentiate between the two main syndromes that cause cognitive decline in dogs due to their old age, both in terms of pathophysiology aspects and the progress of the syndromes, which also complicates their treatment.

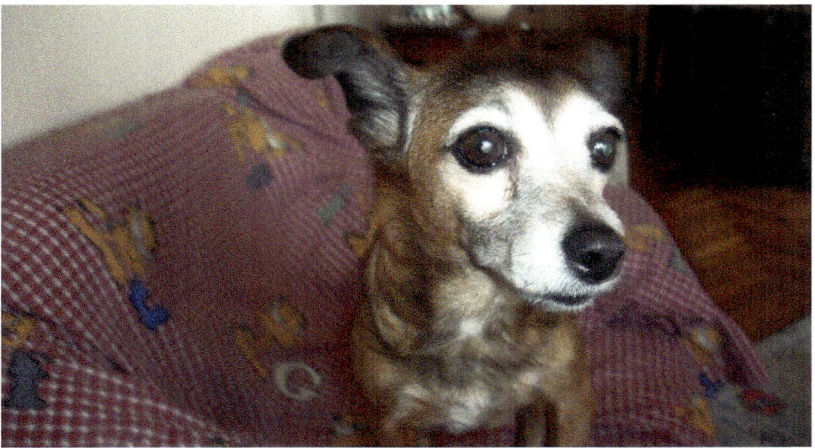

Figure 1. Elderly dogs may suffer from altered sleep–wake cycles and therefore become active at night.

THE ROLE OF OWNERS

The main driving force behind the behavioural changes seen in elderly dogs, regardless of the organic alterations typically associated with old age, is that owners do not always realise their pet has grown old.

This may be because dogs undergo these changes very quickly. Thus, a 12-year-old dog can transform from adulthood to old age in 3–4 months (Fig. 2). In other cases, owners do not realise because their pet still retains some of its active spirit (e.g. chasing cats, mounting females, etc.), which makes them believe the dog is only pretending to be tired.

> Owners who do not realise their dog is now an elderly animal commit the grave mistake of treating it the same way as always.

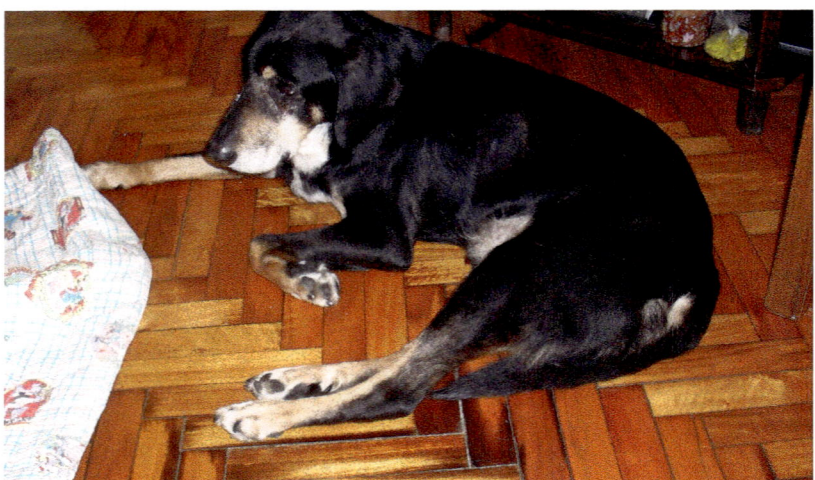

Figure 2. A 12-year-old dog can progress into old age quickly in a few months.

GUIDELINES FOR TREATING ELDERLY DOGS

Elderly dogs need to:

➤ Receive a lot of patience, understanding, and care.

➤ Go for shorter walks or with more stops to rest.

➤ Receive more physical contact: since the dog's sensory functions are in decline, physical contact helps it feel more secure (Fig. 3).

➤ Use collars and leads, even around the home (in the case of very old dogs), as it helps the dog feel guided.

➤ Be allowed to rest for most of the day and only expected to exercise for brief periods.

➤ Receive help to reach the end of their lives with the best possible quality of life.

The vet is responsible for ensuring that the owner understands, accepts, and adapts accordingly to their dog's new circumstances.

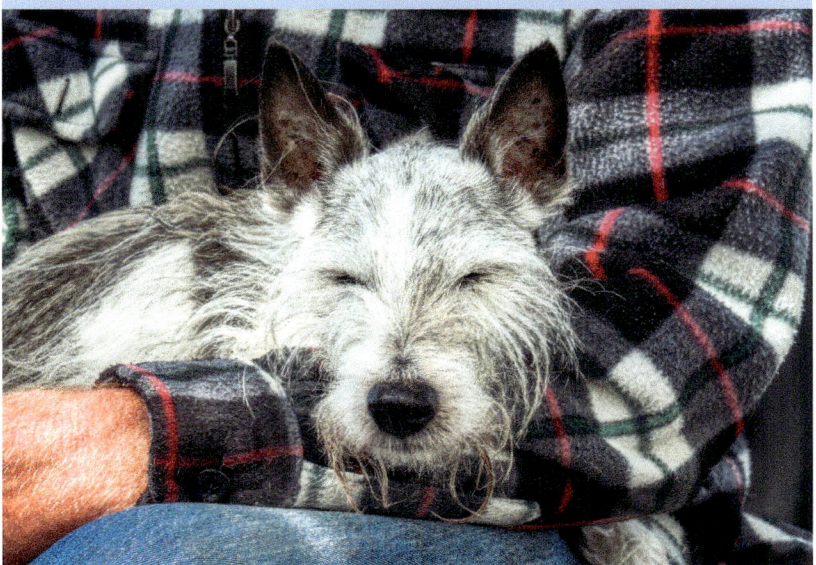

Figure 3. Physical contact helps elderly dogs feel secure.

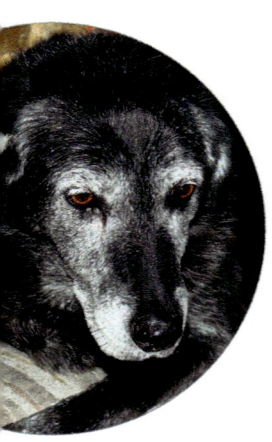

COGNITIVE DYSFUNCTION SYNDROME OR SENILE DEMENTIA

Just like humans, pets suffer a progressive reduction in their cognitive abilities as they advance from adulthood to old age.

> Behavioural disorders in elderly dogs can have several causes, some related to clinical problems and others to the neurochemical changes occurring in the brain due to the ageing process.

Common medical conditions in elderly dogs (intracranial tumours, osteoarthritis, disc diseases, endocrine disorders, etc.) will inevitably lead to negative changes in the animal's behaviour. Dogs become more irritable and consequently more aggressive, or they may suffer from adynamia and apathy. The sensory deterioration typically observed in old age, such as vision loss due to cataracts and deafness, also causes the dog to behave differently (excessive vocalisation, destructive behaviour, elimination in inappropriate locations), generally because of greater anxiety.

If the dog lives with other dogs, all of the aforementioned factors could lead to hierarchical repositioning within the group and therefore produce behavioural changes in both the elderly dog and other group members.

On the other hand, the neurochemical changes that occur in the elderly dog's brain are the cause of cognitive dysfunction syndrome (CDS).

CHANGES IN THE CENTRAL NERVOUS SYSTEM

The changes affecting the CNS in dogs with cognitive dysfunction syndrome are:

➤ An increase in free radicals due to the metabolic breakdown of dead neurons, which is toxic for the remaining healthy neurons (Fig. 4).

➤ A reduction in central dopamine levels due to an increase in monoamine oxidase B activity (MAO-B).

➤ A loss of fluidity in the lipid bilayer of the neuronal synaptic membrane.

Furthermore, other events such as reduced blood flow to the brain and increased blood viscosity will heighten the neurochemical changes.

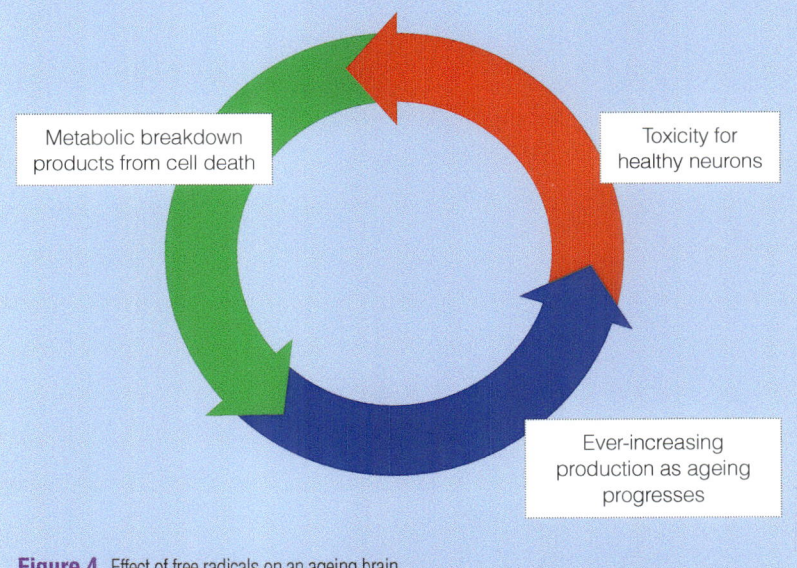

Metabolic breakdown products from cell death

Toxicity for healthy neurons

Ever-increasing production as ageing progresses

Figure 4. Effect of free radicals on an ageing brain.

DIAGNOSIS

The diagnosis should be made according to information collected in the anamnesis and the patient's clinical record, and by direct observation of the patient.

The main changes detected in routine veterinary practice in dogs with CDS are:

➤ Less social interaction: whether with the dog's owners (less playful, less obedient, etc.), with other humans, or with other animals (less interest in positive or negative relationships with other dogs, cats, etc.).

➤ Altered sleep–wake cycle: dogs may walk around at night and sleep during the day.

➤ Temporal and spatial disorientation: dogs with CDS may become disorientated from time to time (Fig. 5).

➤ Loss of hygiene habits with respect to urination and defaecation.

➤ General decline in activity: dogs may not get excited about going for a walk, show no interest in playing, and are often only interested in food; however, by contrast, sometimes they lose their appetite.

➤ Reduced sensory perception: dogs are scared by everyday objects, do not register soft sounds, etc.

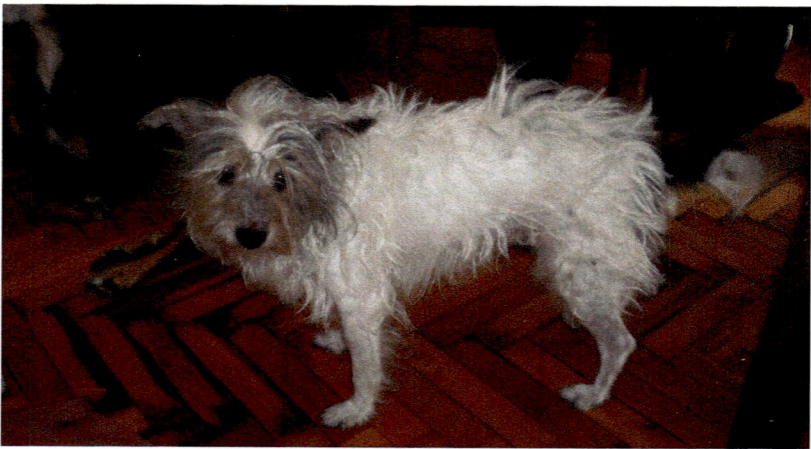

Figure 5. Disorientation is a typical sign of cognitive dysfunction syndrome.

PROGNOSIS

The prognosis is guarded because this behavioural disorder cannot be cured, although there are various therapeutic options that can help alleviate the clinical signs and improve both the patient's and owner's quality of life.

TREATMENT

While CDS is approached using a mixture of pharmacological and behavioural treatments, as are most behavioural alterations, in this case drug therapy is particularly important.

> **The first step is to treat any clinical alterations accordingly before initiating the behavioural therapy.**

- ➤ **Behavioural therapy:** the aim is to change how owners treat and interact with their elderly dog:
  - ➤ Change the owner's attitude: do not force dogs to do certain activities and eliminate any environmental stimuli that affect the patient's behaviour.
  - ➤ Change the patient's environment: leave lights on at night, remove obstacles from areas where the dog paces around, and so on.
  - ➤ Ensure that owners accept their dog's old age and lower their demands placed on their pet.

- ➤ **Drug treatment:** this is designed to minimise the effects of the neurochemical changes that occur in elderly patients. Vets have an arsenal of drugs available to them, which they can use according to their clinical judgement and experience. The main drugs recommended for prescription are:
  - ➤ Citicoline (metabolic neural activator): 25 mg/animal every 12 hours via oral.
  - ➤ Selegiline (MAO-B inhibitor): 2.5 mg/animal every 12 hours taken orally. This reduces dopamine degradation.
  - ➤ Nicergoline (alpha-receptor blocking cerebral vasodilator): 0.25–0.50 mg/kg/day, orally.
  - ➤ Propentofylline (xanthine derivative): 3–5 mg/kg every 12 hours by mouth. It mainly acts by inhibiting adenosine reuptake, thereby increasing its extracellular concentrations; but it also inhibits the phosphodiesterase enzyme which breaks down cyclic-AMP.

PREVENTION

To improve this type of alteration, dogs should be given a suitably enriched and balanced diet, have their cognitive skills stimulated through an enriched environment, and their minds should be kept active (by revising obedience exercises, practising simple games, or using smart toys, etc.) (Fig. 6).

> Ageing is a normal process at the end of any dog's life, so it cannot be avoided.

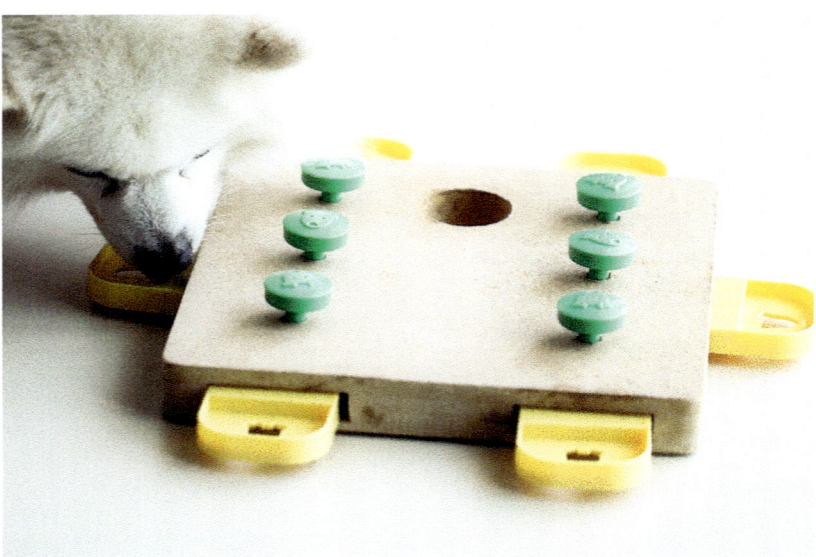

Figure 6. It is essential to keep the dog's mind active to improve the behavioural alterations associated with old age.

ANTIOXIDANTS USED TO PREVENT CDS

Antioxidants such as vitamins E and C, and other substances with cell membrane protective properties, can help prevent CDS. Commercial diets supplemented with these ingredients are now available for elderly dogs.

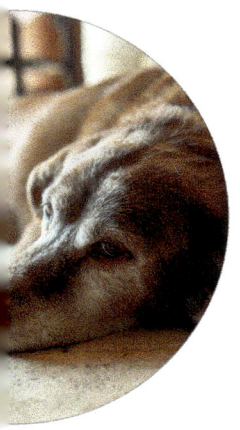

"OLD PUPPY" SYNDROME

All of the foregoing regarding CDS is also applicable in the case of "old puppy" syndrome. The difference lies in the main clinical signs exhibited by the patient, rather than the aetiopathogenesis of the syndromes.

> This syndrome causes the patient's owners a lot of distress, so it is the most common reason for behavioural consultations with respect to elderly dogs in routine practice.

DIAGNOSIS

The diagnosis rests on information gathered during the anamnesis in the consultation. The main indications reported by owners are:

➤ Reduction in the dog's daily activity.
➤ Sleep disorders: dogs wake their owners up because they want to go out at night.
➤ Loss of hygiene habits: elderly dogs develop elimination behaviours similar to the ones they exhibited as puppies, hence the name of the syndrome. Owners find it hard to understand why their dog starts to do things that they have already learnt not to do.

The other signs are those typical of CDS: reduced vigour and attention, lethargy, diminished sensory perception, disorientation to time and space, loss of appetite, hyperattachment, and irritability, amongst others.

PROGNOSIS

The prognosis spans from guarded to good, as it is more favourable than the case of CDS. If the dog's actions that cause the owners the most problems (inappropriate elimination, waking up in the middle of the night, etc.) can be mitigated, then this will restore their good relationship and the owners will be more willing to understand what their pet is going through and to adapt how they manage the situation. This improvement can sometimes lead owners to believe their dog is better, although this is not really the case.

TREATMENT

While there is an even greater arsenal of medications available to treat old puppy syndrome, behavioural therapy is crucial to achieve an overall improvement and restore the positive bond between the patient and its owners.

➤ **Behavioural therapy:**
  ➤ Change the owner's attitude: do not force dogs to do certain activities and eliminate any environmental stimuli that affect the patient's behaviour.
  ➤ Improve the environment: leave lights on at night, remove obstacles from areas where the dog paces around, and so on.
  ➤ Ensure that owners accept their dog's old age and lower their expectations accordingly.
  ➤ Adapt the dog's routine while taking into account the changes it is going through.

➤ **Drug treatment:** the options are similar to CDS, but psychoactive drugs can also be used to reduce or mask the clinical signs that cause the most inconvenience and distress for the owners. Sometimes the vet should change drugs until they determine which generates the best response in the patient and they could even use combinations.
  ➤ Citicoline (metabolic neural activator): 25 mg/animal every 12 hours, orally.
  ➤ Selegiline (MAO-B inhibitor): 2.5 mg/animal every 12 hours taken orally. This reduces dopamine degradation.
  ➤ Nicergoline (alpha-receptor blocking cerebral vasodilator): 0.25–0.50 mg/kg/day, orally.
  ➤ Propentofylline (xanthine derivative): 3–5 mg/kg every 12 hours, orally.
  ➤ Buspirone 2.5–10 mg/animal/day split over two oral doses. Buspirone has a broad therapeutic range and provokes a good anxiolytic response.
  ➤ Fluoxetine (SSRI): 0.5–1 mg/kg/day in a single oral dose.
  ➤ Paroxetine (SSRI): 0.5–1 mg/kg/day in a single oral dose.
  ➤ Clomipramine (tricyclic antidepressant): 1.0–3.0 mg/kg/day given orally in 2 doses. This drug has significant SSRI-like activity.

PREVENTION

Constant, moderate mental stimulation and physical exercise are very effective preventive measures (e.g. revisiting obedience exercises, simple games, etc.).

As with cognitive dysfunction syndrome, the administration of antioxidants, such as vitamins E and C, and other substances with cell membrane protective properties, prevent the behavioural alterations associated with old puppy syndrome.

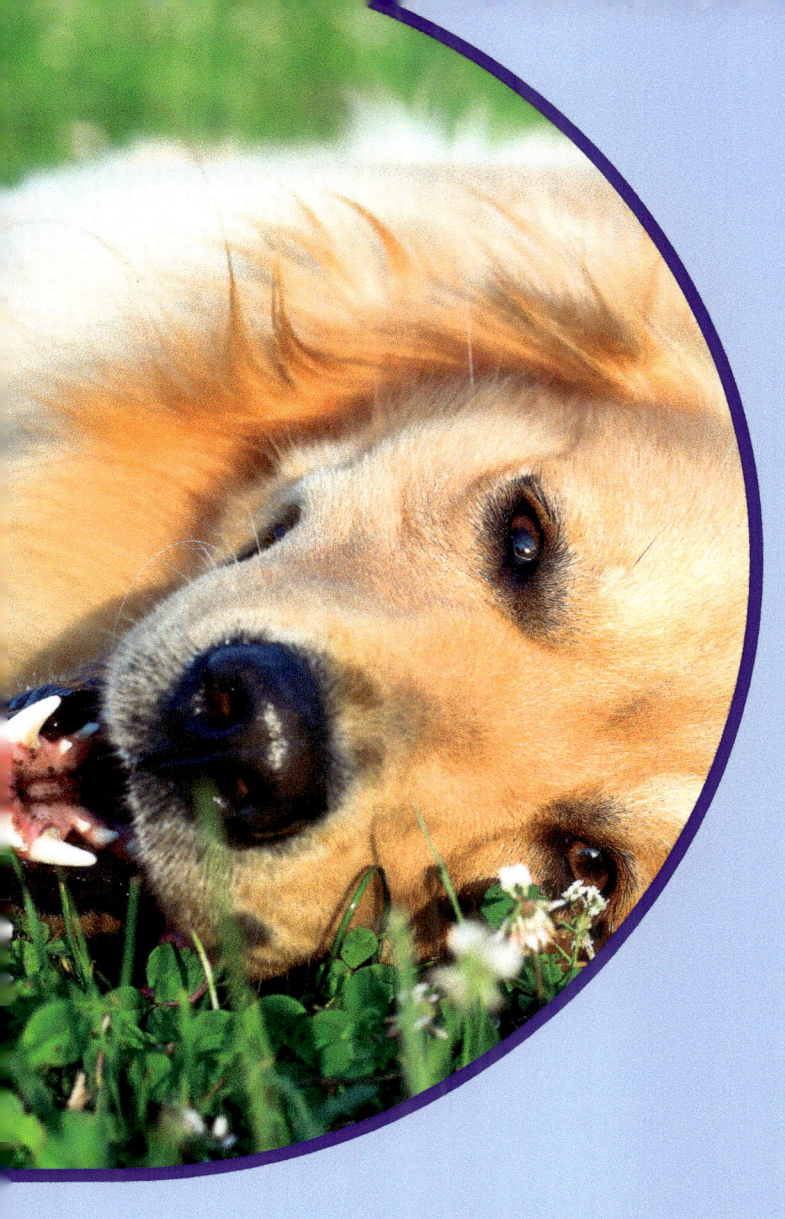

LATEST TREATMENT ADVANCES AND INNOVATIONS

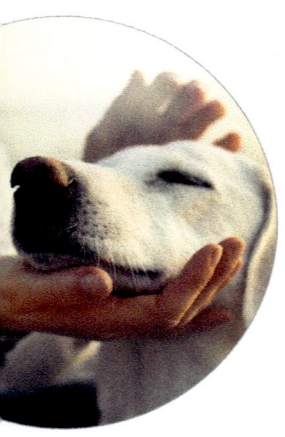

INTRODUCTION

Currently, we are undoubtedly seeing some significant and rapid changes in many different disciplines. Veterinary medicine forms part of this panorama, so these advances also include the study of animal behaviour or ethology. One of the most evolving areas of ethology is, in fact, the development of new treatments for dogs with behavioural disorders.

This chapter deals with some of the most relevant new therapies.

DOG PHEROMONES

Dog pheromones have seen a recent increase in popularity as aids in the treatment of behavioural alterations in pet dogs, although they have not reached the same levels as cat pheromones.

Obviously, dog pheromones have the same mechanism of action as their feline equivalents. Pheromones are chemicals secreted by animals that produce predictable effects on the behaviour of the individual that receives them, provided that both animals belong to the same species. They are closely related to the olfactory system and CNS, and fulfil an important function in a dog's communicative and social behaviour (Fig. 1).

The main natural sources of canine pheromones are vaginal exudates, urine, and secretions from skin glands, both sebaceous and apocrine sweat glands, located in the head, perineal area, and interdigital spaces.

> Pheromones affect sexual, social, and territorial behaviours in individual animals.

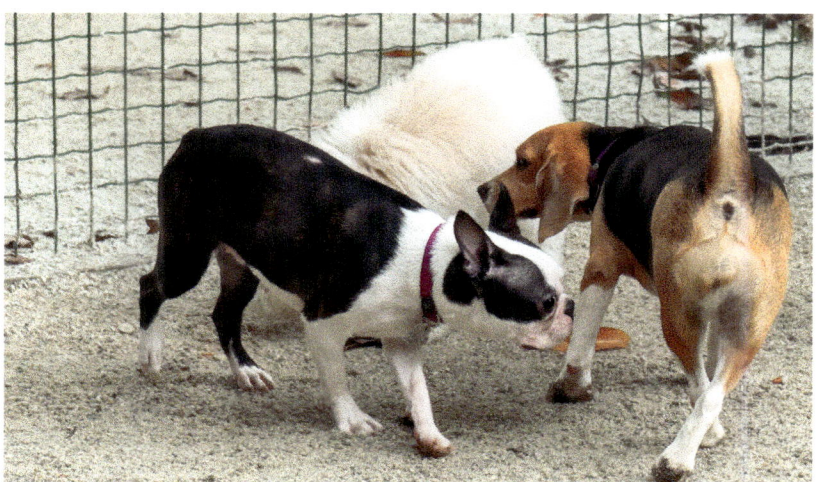

Figure 1. Pheromones play an essential role in communication between dogs.

THE VOMERONASAL ORGAN OR JACOBSON'S ORGAN

The vomeronasal organ, or Jacobson's organ, forms part of a dog's olfactory system and is heavily involved in the mechanism of action of canine pheromones. It is located on the vomer bone, between the nose and mouth, just above the dog's upper canine teeth (Fig. 2). It has olfactory nerve endings that differ from those found in the nose. These nerve pathways carry additional information to the cortical olfactory centre. It is a secondary system that helps when the animal cannot definitively identify an odour and corresponds to a crucial link in pheromones' mechanism of action.

Figure 2. Sagittal view of the cranium of a dog showing the locations of the vomeronasal organ and olfactory centre.

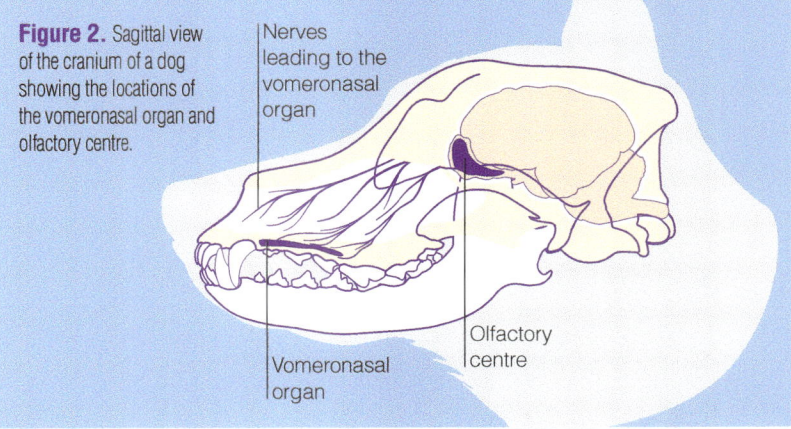

Nerves leading to the vomeronasal organ

Olfactory centre

Vomeronasal organ

PHEROMONE CLASSIFICATION

Depending on their **mode of action** and **effects**, pheromones are classified as:

➤ Primer pheromones: produce slow and enduring changes in the recipient's reproductive physiological.
➤ Releaser pheromones: produce immediate but short-lived changes in the recipient. These pheromones generate a sense of wellbeing and calm in the recipient.

Depending on their **chemical composition**, pheromones are classed as:

➤ Volatile pheromones: these are releaser pheromones captured in the olfactory mucosa.
➤ Nonvolatile pheromones: these are primer pheromones which seem to be captured by the vomeronasal organ.

Depending on their **function** from a behavioural perspective, pheromones can be classified as:

➤ Social pheromones: help identify the individual members within a social group. Dogs use pheromones to mark objects or individuals that form part of their familiar environment by rubbing their body against them to generate a feeling of wellbeing, calm, and security. This behaviour is more important and more common in cats.
➤ Sex pheromones: are excreted along with sexual secretions and urine in order to establish contact and approximation with a member of the opposite sex for mating purposes.
➤ Territorial pheromones: are released through urine and from interdigital glands in the paws. As the name suggests, they are used to mark territory.
➤ Alarm pheromones: are secreted from anal glands or sweat glands in the paw pads. They are released in stressful situations whenever the dog is stressed or scared.
➤ Appeasing pheromones: are released by nursing mothers to make their puppies feel relaxed and secure.

Pheromones are not used as a therapeutic tool for dogs as much as they are in cats, but they are still a good option to support the treatment of behavioural disorders.

They are available in different formats (sprays, diffusers, or collars) and their main function is reduce to a dog's stress and anxiety regardless of the stimulus.

> Pheromones should always be used in combination with the corresponding drug and behavioural therapies, as befits each case.

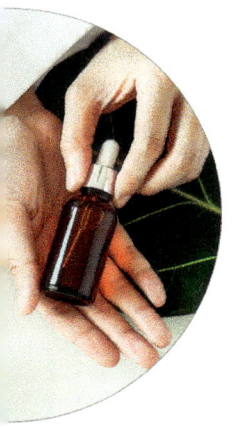

OTHER TREATMENT OPTIONS

Some new therapeutic options have appeared recently that are primarily based on natural compounds. While all medicines, including psychoactive agents, are to some extent derivatives of natural products, society currently favours products that are not widely recognised as psychoactive medicines. The veterinary sector has reacted accordingly to this change and started to produce drugs in line with this tendency.

NATURAL MEDICINES

Essentially, these are medications that incorporate ingredients found in nature. They are based on a blend of plant extracts combined with different vitamins and amino acids.

Given the importance of serotonin, it makes sense that any new products contain some essential amino acids or neurotransmitters (such as γ-amino-butyric acid [GABA]), antioxidants, and plant extracts which have historically helped subjects relax.

> These products are available as oral tablets or drops and indicated as a prophylaxis before stressful situations.

More complex drugs, which incorporate coenzymes such as coenzyme Q10 in addition to antioxidants, vitamins, minerals, amino acids, and mitochondrial cofactors, can be used to treat elderly animals with cognitive dysfunction.

There are also products based on a combination of L-theanine and L-tryptophan with plant extracts (such as *Piper methysticum* extracts) and B vitamins that act on the central nervous system. They are available as tablets for oral administration.

Some of the natural compounds with the greatest capacity to influence the behaviour of pet dogs, which are often found in the ingredients of natural medicines used as adjuvants in the treatment of behavioural disorders, include:

THEANINE

L-Theanine is an amino acid found in green tea (Fig. 3). While the molecule is not actually a sedative, it is responsible for the calming and relaxing effects associated with green tea. This is because it increases GABA levels, reduces glutamate neurotoxicity, and has a positive effect on serotonin levels.

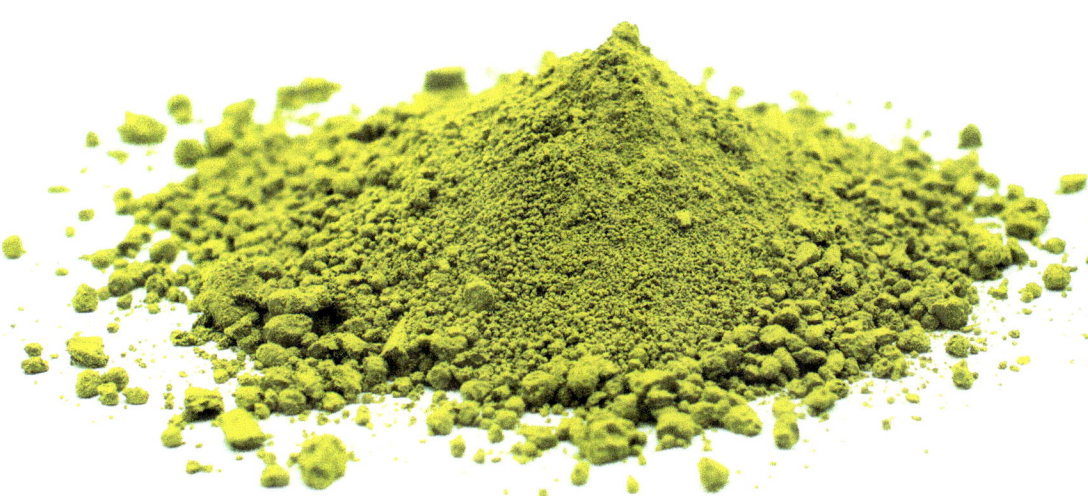

Figure 3. Matcha tea contains up to five times more L-theanine than green tea.

TRYPTOPHAN

Tryptophan is an essential amino acid that dogs can only obtain through their diet.

The amino acid L-tryptophan is the metabolic precursor of serotonin, a neurotransmitter that plays a vital role in the regulation of anxiety, appetite, and sleep. Once the body has absorbed L-tryptophan, tryptophan hydroxylase (the rate-limiting enzyme in serotonin biosynthesis) converts it into L-5-hydroxytryptophan, which is then transformed into 5-hydroxytryptamine or serotonin by decarboxylase.

Tryptophan must cross the blood–brain barrier before it can exert its effect; however, it has to compete with long-chain neutral amino acids (tyrosine, phenylalanine, valine, leucine, and isoleucine) that use the same transporters. Tryptophan-rich diets can induce a calming effect in aggressive dogs and tryptophan supplements may increase the feeling of wellbeing in some patients.

> Balanced diets with tryptophan and long-chain neutral amino acids have been shown to improve the signs of anxiety and, therefore, abnormal behaviour in dogs.

VITAMIN B$_3$

Vitamin B$_3$ is water soluble and easily added to the diet. It affects metabolism by acting as the prosthetic group in coenzymes or as a coenzyme precursor. Vitamin B$_3$ takes on two main forms, niacin (nicotinic acid) and its amide form, nicotinamide.

> Nicotinamide has a very similar physiological action on the central nervous system as the anxiolytic effects of benzodiazepines.

α-CASOZEPINE

Several studies have investigated the use of α-casozepine in dogs with anxiety.

α-Casozepine is a milk casein derivative (the α-S1-casein fraction), in this case, of bovine origin. It is available as tablets for oral administration, but it can also be incorporated as an ingredient in food.

In nursing puppies, trypsin is the enzyme responsible for hydrolysing casein in their mother's milk into α-casozepine, which binds with GABA receptors in the brain and produces a calming effect similar to that of diazepam, but without its side effects (sedation, lack of inhibition, and addiction). Dogs tolerate this natural relaxant very well, whether in its purest form, a supplement, or a food ingredient.

As puppies grow, their digestive system changes and tends to hydrolyse pepsin instead of casein, so adult dogs only produce very small amounts of α-casozepine.

> α-Casozepine has been used with good results to treat anxiety and stress-related symptoms.

α-Casozepine has a selective affinity for the benzodiazepine binding site in $GABA_A$ receptors in the brain, thus enhancing the effects of GABA, a neurotransmitter that is well-known for its ability to inhibit anxiety and stress-related disorders.

When α-casozepine attaches to its specific binding site on the GABA receptor, it can increase GABA's affinity for its own neurorecepter. This increases the opening frequency of the associated chloride ion channels, resulting in GABA-induced hyperpolarisation of the axonal membrane and subsequently a reduction in the brain's postsynaptic neuronal activity. This enhances the inhibitory action of any available GABA and produces an anxiolytic effect.

α-Casozepine was compared to an anxiolytic control (selegiline) for the treatment of anxiety disorders in dogs in a 2007 study published in the Journal of Veterinary Behavior and the results revealed promising efficacy.

> α-Casozepine aids in the prevention of anxiety in foreseeable stressful situations such as moving home, the arrival of a baby, changes in the owner's routine, visits to the vet, and so on.

α-Casozepine is safe for both cats and dogs and there are no known side effects to date. Nor does it have any contraindications.

NUTRACEUTICALS

Nutraceuticals are functional foods that help improve a patient's quality of life, keep them in good health, and prevent diseases. As such, foods enriched with vitamins and minerals, or which contain modified ingredients (fatty acids, fibre, etc.), can be considered nutraceutical products.

The range of veterinary products available includes different types of functional foods indicated for certain behavioural alterations (aggression, anxiety, stress, etc.). These products comprise natural ingredients, like those mentioned earlier, which dogs incorporate into the body through their diet.

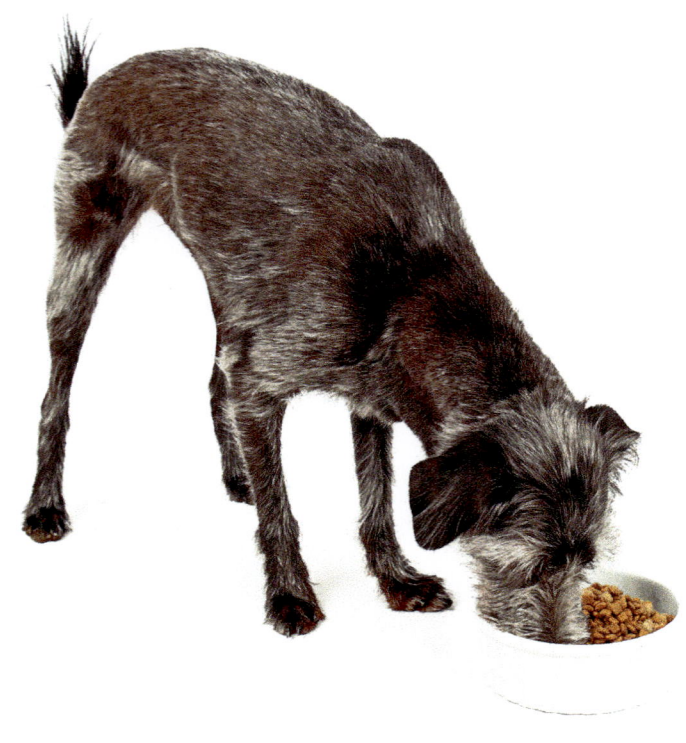

THE IMPORTANCE OF PROACTIVE OWNER PARTICIPATION

Complementary therapies can form a very useful part of therapeutic strategies to address behavioural disorders in dogs, but they do not represent an ideal treatment by themselves. This is because when it comes to resolving behavioural disorders, it is the patient's owner who must proactively participate by implementing the environmental changes and behaviour modification techniques indicated by the veterinary specialist.

An essential element of a successful treatment is to convince owners of the importance of their active participation and to avoid the misconception that medications or a specific diet will suffice.

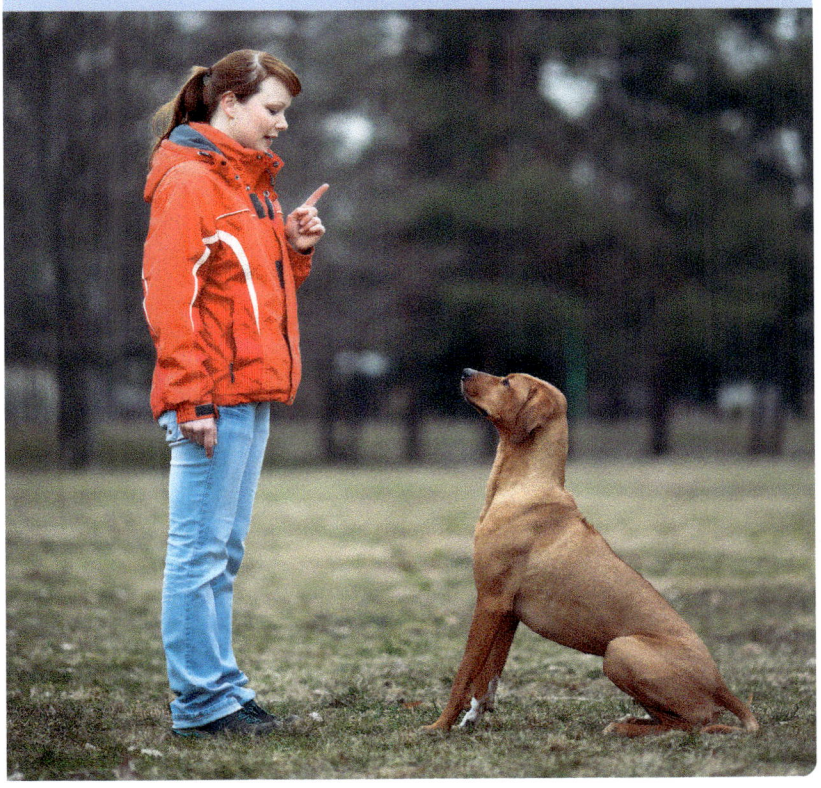

BEHAVIOURAL DISORDERS
IN CATS

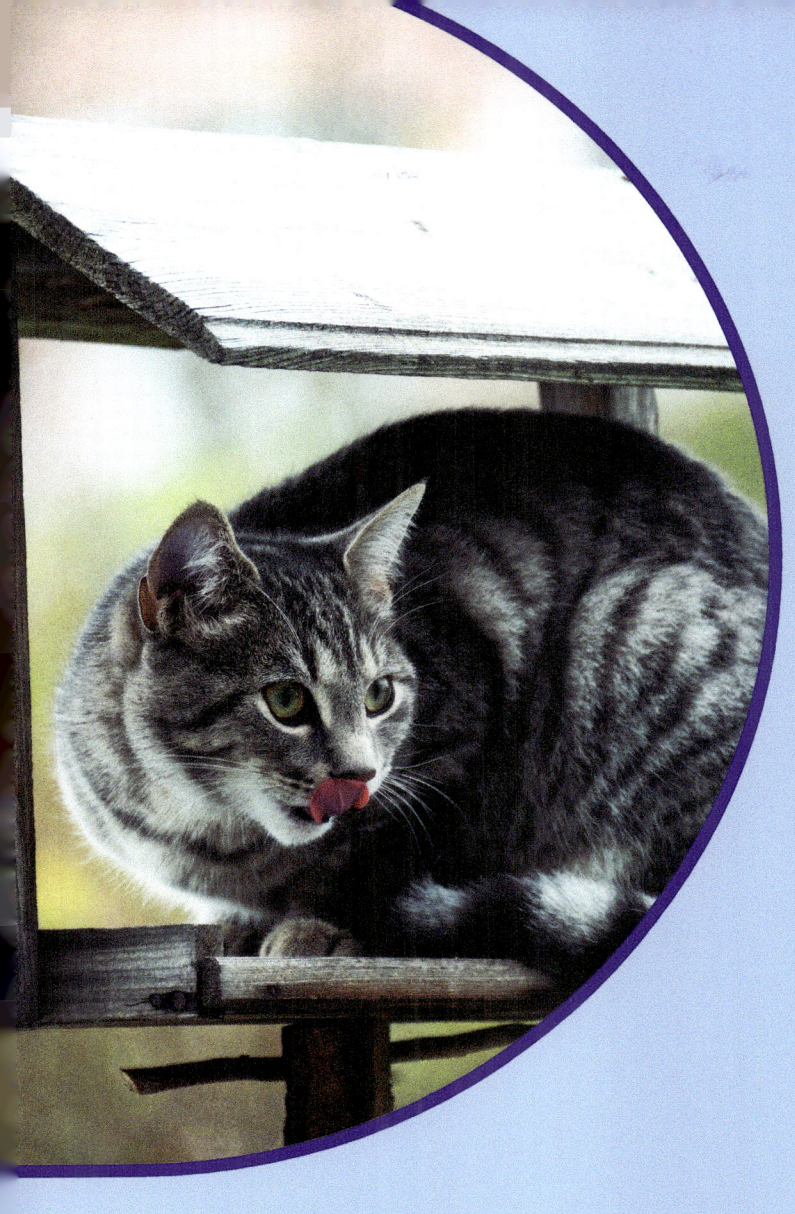

READ ME FIRST

BEHAVIOURAL DISORDERS IN CATS

Humans have only been able to confine one animal as a household pet without letting it walk on the grass, climb a tree, or try to hunt its prey. We are talking about cats.

As veterinary medicine has advanced and the risks of injuries and diseases have become apparent, more and more cat lovers have recommended permanent and rigorous indoor confinement as a preventive health measure.

However, this relatively recent confinement, which has developed over the last 50 years or so, goes against cats' independent nature. The reduction in the species' freedom has occurred in parallel with a huge increase in urbanisation and the growth of large cities, during which time pets have assumed a new role, particularly cats, to help cover the emotional shortcomings that are so common among urban dwellers. Before we can appreciate how this captivity is partly responsible for the onset of behavioural problems in strictly indoor cats, we must first understand the intimate nature inherent to cats as a species.

The earliest recognised ancestor of cats were the miacids. These small carnivores inhabited the earth millions of years ago and were the common predecessor of felines and canines (Fig. 1). Yet evidence of cats, similar to the ones we know and love today, only goes back some 8,000–10,000 years, while they were first domesticated in ancient Egypt about 3,000–5,000 years ago (Fig. 2).

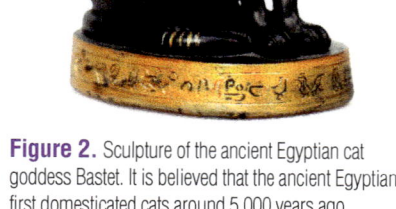

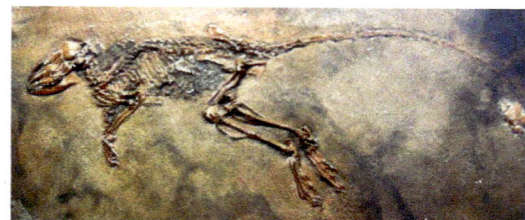

Figure 1. Fossil of a miacid, the common ancestor of cats and dogs.

Figure 2. Sculpture of the ancient Egyptian cat goddess Bastet. It is believed that the ancient Egyptians first domesticated cats around 5,000 years ago.

The cat species domesticated itself for its own benefit, as both waste food produced by humans and the rodents attracted to human settlements were a readily available source of food (Fig. 3). This is why cats quickly learnt to live in close contact with humans, which demonstrates their incredible adaptability.

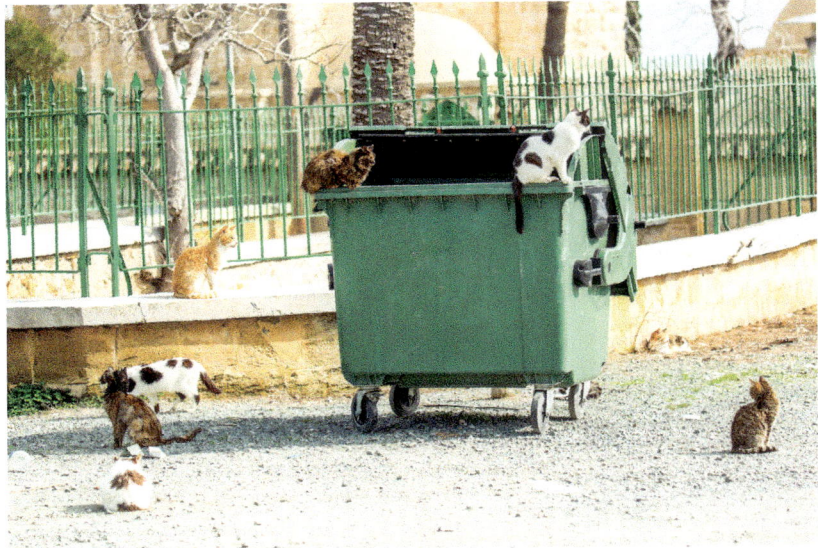

Figure 3. Street cats looking for food in rubbish containers.

Humans have domesticated other species for our own benefit, but this was not the case with cats. While it is true that humans have genetically modified cats, mainly for aesthetic reasons, we have not applied selective breeding to alter their function as in the case of dogs, for example.

Cats are self-sufficient and can return to their ancestral and innate survival instincts quickly and without any difficulties. They need four basic skills to ensure their survival: hunting, feeding, reproduction, and rearing offspring. The strong, instinctive traits so typical of cats have evolved over millennia to fulfil these requirements to perfection.

BEHAVIOURAL DISORDERS IN CATS

Cats are carnivorous predators. They hunt small prey and mostly at night (they are nocturnal), which reduces their exposure to their own predators and therefore their vulnerability. They are solitary predators and do not form social groups for hunting or to provide protection. Females are very maternal (Fig. 4) and raise their offspring to be self-sufficient in a short period, before resources for the population's growth are depleted. This makes cats very territorial, and their territory must be defined and defended from any intruding cats that may compete for such resources.

> The five characteristic traits of cats are: predatory, nocturnal, solitary, maternal, and territorial.

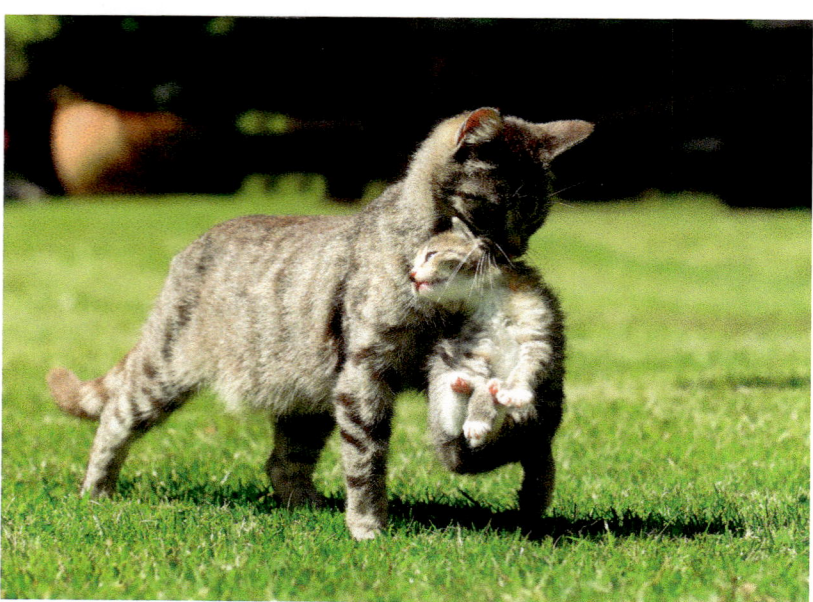

Figure 4. Cats tend to be very maternal.

Humans have clearly changed the natural living conditions for their pet cats based on the assumption that our definition of a good life is an improvement for them.

When in its natural environment, the search for food takes up a large part of a cat's daily activity. Given that cats hunt alone, it is reasonable to assume that they do no wait until they are hungry before looking for their next meal. As solitary predators, cats must constantly be on the prowl to catch their sustenance long before the physiological need arises. Many hunts have to be aborted or fail for various reasons. Cats may hunt for hours, even days, before catching an acceptable prey. Pet cats kept indoors since they were kittens experience a decline in their instinctive need to hunt, since their food is guaranteed, and they are often given too much. Shortly after weaning, the mother will teach her litter to take responsibility for feeding themselves, but in the case of pets, the owner takes over this educational role and teaches the kittens what and how to eat. Cats learn quickly, which is only natural, and their human companions soon become their surrogate mothers.

Although cats are solitary by nature, they are not antisocial, but instead amazingly and wonderfully independent. Domestic cats look to form part of a social group but while always maintaining their independence. In a natural setting, female adults delimit a territory that is large enough to provide security and food for themselves and their offspring. Potential mates can only enter the female's domain during oestrus. Mother cats must quickly train their kittens to be self-sufficient hunters before puberty brings them additional problems or resources are exhausted by the litter's growing demands. Consequently, mothers spend a lot of time protecting their territory and offspring, hunting for food, and teaching their young. Although we often believe that male cats are territorial, it is actually the females who are more possessive of their own ground, much more reluctant to accept intruders (real or perceived), and far less tolerant of being forced to accept another cat in their territory. However, proximity to humans drastically increased the availability of food and therefore kittens could mature, reproduce, and remain in social colonies for the rest of their lives.

BEHAVIOURAL DISORDERS IN CATS

Considering what makes a cat a cat, we have to ask ourselves, what are the possible consequences of imposing our lifestyle on our cats? Based on recommendations from the veterinary profession, and to better accommodate what most people want, pets are often sterilised at a very young age. This eliminates the time they would have spent courting, mating, gestating, and rearing kittens. We also provide food for our cats, which eradicates any need to hunt. When young cats are at an impressionable age (period of socialisation), we not only teach them that tasty, high-calorie foods are always available in unlimited amounts, but also that, besides eating, their lives will not involve any meaningful activities. Cats that live alone will spend most of their time waiting for brief moments of companionship with their busy owners. Cats living in a household with other cats, on the other hand, can only hope that they have amenable housemates rather than a herd or pack imposed by a well-meaning cat lover. This is because, like it or not, they are enclosed in a confined space for their entire lives. And when a cat dislikes its situation and feels uncomfortable it may resort to hunting or stalking humans, attacking its imposed feline housemates, inappropriate elimination in locations other than in its litter box, and so on. This is when we recognise that the cat has a behavioural problem and try to alleviate its stress by means of antidepressants or other medications.

As a profession, perhaps we should reconsider the advice we give to cat owners in light of the consequences of their pets' inactivity and sedentary lifestyle, which includes a growing list of diseases associated with and triggered by stress.

Cats with outdoor access spend most of their time climbing, exploring, marking their territory, observing, waiting, stalking, hunting, and feeding themselves. They also decide who may or may not enter their social circle. However, it is also true that they could suffer a serious injury, come into contact with parasites and diseases (including potentially fatal ones), and would be exposed to dangers.

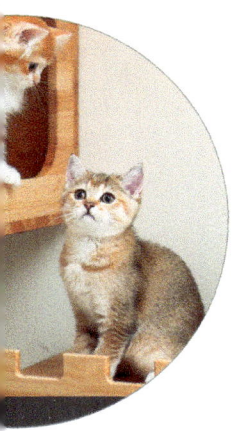

ENVIRONMENTAL ENRICHMENT

Owners should always be encouraged to enrich their cat's home environment. Exterior enclosures can offer indoor cats safe access to outdoor spaces. These enclosures could be small, cheap, and discreet areas or relatively large like an extension to the main house. Anyone, from people living in flats with a window or balcony to owners of spacious houses, can provide their cat access to an open-air area. If an exterior space is available, fencing or nets represent a cheap but safe means of allowing cats contact with a natural environment where they can climb trees, hide behind bushes, stretch out in the sun, or explore a lawn. When there is only limited or no outdoor access, the indoor environment can be improved by introducing entertainment and stimulation for cats that live alone or respite for cats that share their home with other cats. From a very early age, cages can be used to define each cat's personal territory. A simple training technique to persuade cats to use cages consists of placing young cats in a cage large enough to cover all their needs: food, water, litter tray, and sleeping area. It should also include toys or an area where they can climb and hide. When the owner is home, the kitten should be let out of its cage to explore and make use of the entire house, and to interact with the owner. Over time, the cage can be left open for increasingly longer periods until eventually it is open permanently and the animal can move around freely. Since the cat can meet all of its needs inside the cage, it will start to recognise this small area as its own territory; this instils a feeling of security. Climbing towers and shelves on walls make great areas for cats to exercise and they help preserve social order. Commercially available trees and furniture for cats usually feature several areas where they can climb, hide, and occupy individual platforms. Placing these structures close to a window also presents further advantages (Fig. 5). It is a good idea to hide food in different locations to entertain the cat by simulating hunting. This trick also constrains how much it eats better than a tray full of food.

> As veterinary professionals, we have to accept the lifestyle that our clients establish for their cats, but we also have an obligation to advise them about the best options for their pet's health and wellbeing.

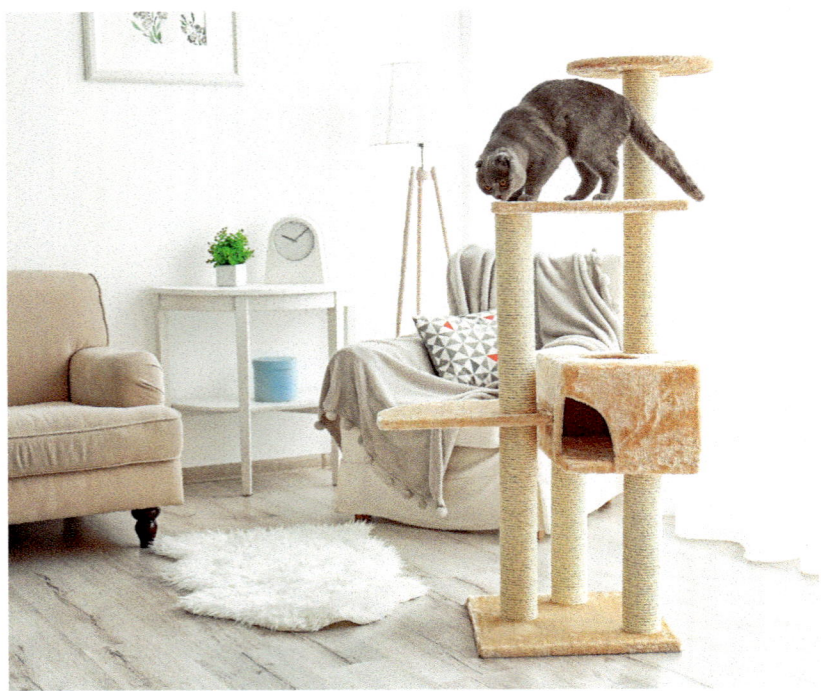

Figure 5. An example of environmental enrichment.

BASIC RECOMMENDATIONS

➤ Insofar as possible, house cats should be permitted to live an independent life and set out their own periods of activity. For example, when a cat approaches its owner for contact, they should play with it, but always by means of a toy that acts an intermediary between the animal and its owner, and when the cat wishes to distance itself, it should be allowed to do so.

➤ Owners should never use their hands as a toy when playing with their cats. They should also let them doze as much as they want. Remember cats generally become active when it starts to get dark, as their circadian rhythm (the body's internal corticosteroid secretion cycle) is opposite to that of humans and dogs.

➤ They eat and drink small amounts several times a day, so their bowl should be filled daily, and they should be allowed to regulate their own feeding. However, be careful not to overfeed them.

➤ The litter box should be located in a quiet area with very few passers-by (not in a hallway) and filled with a material that the cat seems to like.

➤ Owners should not let anyone annoy their cat (particularly bored children and teenagers). What is more, house cats can turn aggressive towards people.

➤ Castrating males reduces their propensity to act aggressively, become vagrants, and softens the distinctive pungent smell of their urine. In females, castration prevents the possibility of the animal developing any reproductive system diseases. Another clear benefit of castration in both sexes is to prevent indiscriminate reproduction.

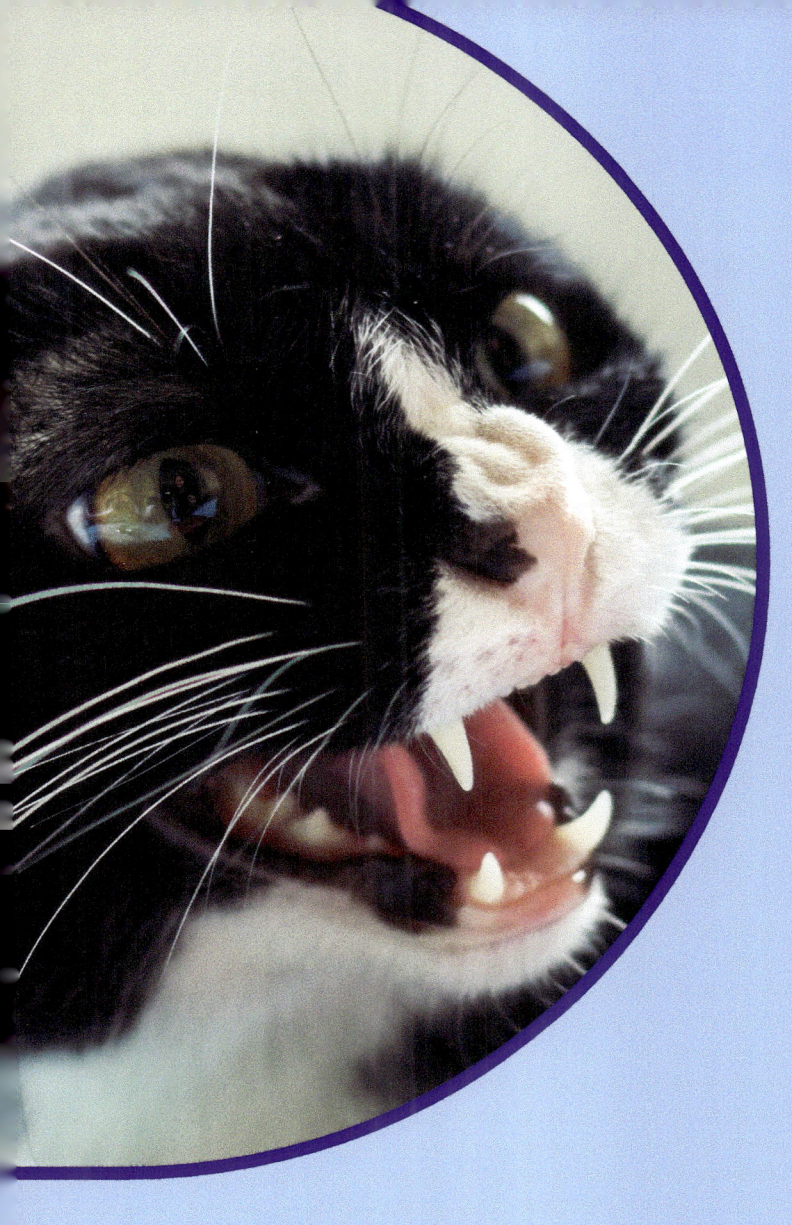

DISORDERS ASSOCIATED WITH AGGRESSIVE BEHAVIOUR

INTRODUCTION

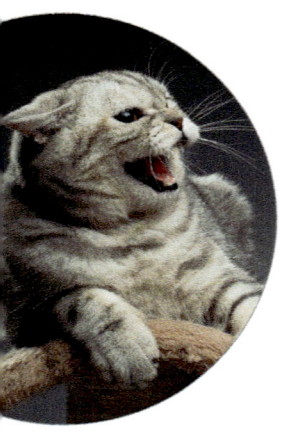

Animal behaviour specialists view felines, that is, all members of the Felidae family, as ideal predators, since both their bodies and minds are perfectly developed and adapted for hunting. As a member of the feline family, this consideration also applies to the domestic cat.

THE HUNTING CAT

The main characteristics of cats as hunters are:

➤ Solitary.
➤ Primarily nocturnal.
➤ They hunt prey that are smaller than themselves, mainly rodents but also, to a lesser degree, small birds.
➤ They tend to hunt in open ground and tall pastures, and their technique involves hiding, waiting, and ambushing their victims.
➤ Cats do not stalk their prey.
➤ They do not share their prey with their fellow cats, except for the case of mothers with their kittens.

Besides their athletic muscles, phenomenal agility, and exceptional night vision, house cats have become excellent hunters thanks to some of their special anatomical adaptations. For example, although the lower jaw has a very limited range of lateral movement, its anatomy has evolved so that it functions as a lever when the cat applies the fatal bite to any prey it has just captured. This killer bite is also reinforced by the cat's canine teeth that have evolved to possess the ideal curvature to enter the intervertebral space of the victim's neck, thereby severing the spinal cord and immobilising their prey, which protects it from the quarry's defensive attacks. Another anatomical adaptation of note is that cats have a relatively short digestive tract. This means they digest their food quickly, which is why domestic cats follow a dietary pattern of eating small amounts several times a day.

With specific regard to their predatory behavioural patterns, it is worth high-lighting that a cat's hunting behaviour is triggered by the prey's movement, which evokes stalking and eventually the short sprint, pounce, and capture with their claws on their forelimbs, before the lethal bite. From this point on a different, but complementary, behaviour starts – ingestion (eating the prey).

Cats' hunting behaviour has both innate and learned components. Kittens with a hunting mother that live in an almost natural habitat generally learn to hunt when they are 6–20 weeks old and become much more skilful hunters than young cats that do not receive this parental training.

All this information can help us understand why kittens follow their owners' ankles as they pass by; it is not because they are crazy, but rather they are trying to adapt their genetics to their environment. For example, when a cat looks at a pigeon through the window and swishes the tip of its tail ener-getically while grinding its teeth, it is not relishing the possibility of killing the poor bird, it is really suffering internal conflict between what its instinct tells it do and what it can actually do (Fig. 1). It also helps us understand our feline friends when they do not want to accept another cat in the house, their need to exercise their extraordinary muscles, and the huge efforts they have to make to live inside a flat or house.

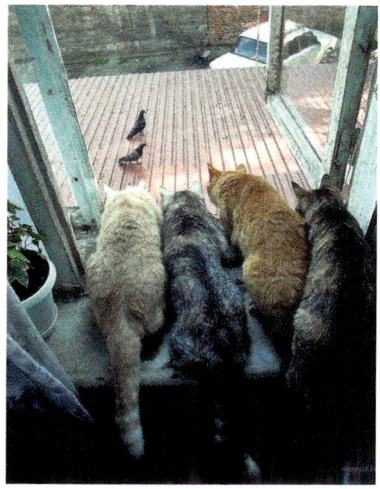

Figure 1. Cats are natural hunters, so they present predatory behavioural patterns.

PATHOPHYSIOLOGY

Researchers in experimental neurology and neuroscience have recently discovered which areas of the brain correspond to the neurological basis or substrate of aggressive behaviour.

The brain structures generally associated with aggression are collectively called the limbic system. This region of the brain, also known as the visceral or reptilian brain or archicerebellum, is considered a primitive structure in comparison with the dense layer of cells called grey matter, neocortex, or neocerebellum.

The limbic system forms a ring around the inner surface of the brain, the anterior inferior portion of which is known as the amygdala or amygdaloid body.

The amygdala is located deep inside each temporal lobe and has been strongly linked to aggressive behaviour. We know that when certain areas of the brain are stimulated it evokes a violent or aggressive response regardless of the situation, context, or subject's prior experience, so these areas constitute the neuronal basis or substrate of aggression.

> The cerebral cortex acts on the hypothalamus and limbic system (amygdala), in turn, these structures affect the midbrain, which brings about the end result – the animal exhibits aggressive behaviour.

Experimental studies have shown that electrical stimulation of the dorsal hypothalamic area elicits defensive behaviour, stimulation of the medial hypothalamus induces offensive behaviour, and, lastly, a controlled electrical discharge on the lateral hypothalamus triggers a predatory conduct in the test animal.

With regard to the influence of neurotransmitters, dopamine, norepinephrine, and acetylcholine all stimulate aggression, whereas serotonin produces an inhibitory effect. The dopaminergic and norepinephrine systems seem to facilitate aggressive behaviour (Fig. 2).

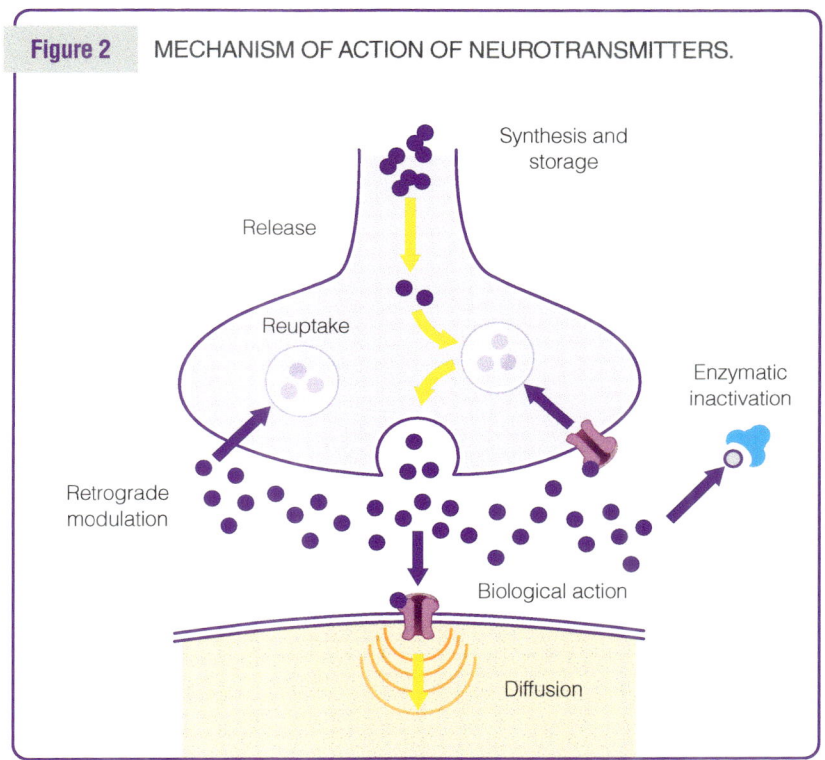

Figure 2 MECHANISM OF ACTION OF NEUROTRANSMITTERS.

Hormones also play an important role in controlling conducts associated with aggression. We now know that androgens increase offensive aggression but have no effect on defensive aggression.

Although apparently counterintuitive, there is no clear evidence of a correlation between high androgen plasma levels and aggressiveness. Male hormones are believed to have an organisational rather than excitatory effect on intrasexual and competitive aggression (both offensive types of aggression). Finally, prolactin is known to contribute to maternal aggression in females.

Aggression-related problems are the most common reason for consultations due to behavioural alterations in dogs and the second leading cause in cats. However, these consultations do not always correspond specifically to a change in the animal's aggressiveness. For example, is it an act of aggression if a dog bites another dog because it feels threatened? Is an animal that growls and bares its teeth at strangers being pathologically aggressive? If a cat extends its claws and raises it hackles in anticipation of a medical examination, does this mean it suffers from a clinical behavioural problem? Should acts of predatory aggression be considered aggressive behaviour?

The answers to these questions depend on different lines of research and prior experience. Despite the complexity of the subject, as with other behavioural alterations, abnormal aggressive behaviour in pets is defined as an impairment to pleasant, harmonious cohabitation with their owners, irrespective of the cause of the alteration (genetic, environmental, etc.) or whether it affects the animal's quality of life or that of its cohabitants.

There is no straightforward or specific definition of aggression; some researchers into human behaviour define it in terms of harmful acts without taking into account aggressive intentions (gestures and postures), some consider that these threatening signals alone constitute an aggressive act, while others, in perhaps the most practical approach, discuss agonistic behaviour, in an adept attempt to circumnavigate the term aggression.

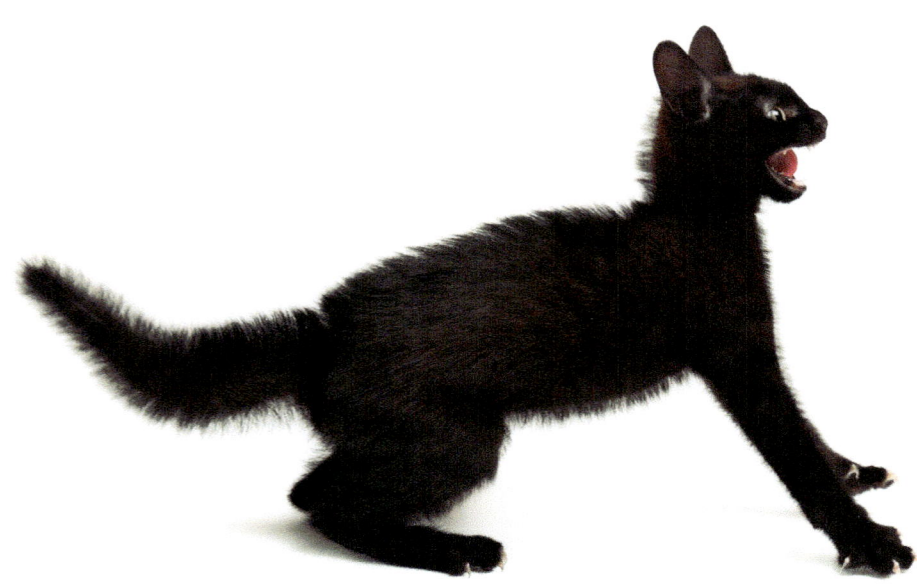

CLASSIFICATION OF AGGRESSION IN CATS

To understand the concept of aggressiveness, we need to learn about the different means of classifying aggression.

BASED ON NERVE STRUCTURES

When certain parts of the brain are stimulated, it gives rise to violent or aggressive conduct regardless of the situation, context, or the individual's previous experiences:

➤ Electrical stimulation of the dorsal hypothalamus causes the animal to exhibit defensive aggressive behaviour.

➤ Electrical stimulation of the medial hypothalamus triggers offensive aggression.

➤ While electrical stimulation of the lateral hypothalamus makes the subject exhibit predatory aggression.

Drawing on these findings, aggressive behaviour has been classified as:

➤ **Affective aggression (social or agonistic):** cats that exhibit this conduct are reluctant to do so; in other words, they do not enjoy behaving in such a manner. It can involve either offensive or defensive actions.

➤ **Nonaffective aggression (predatory):** cats feel gratification from this type of conduct. As such, the animal's behaviour is reinforced, and it is therefore much harder to eradicate these conducts compared to affective aggression.

BASED ON THE SITUATION OR STIMULUS THAT ELICITS THE AGGRESSION

Various types of aggressiveness have been observed among animals. The following classification, one of the most popular, is based on the situation or stimulus that evokes the behaviour:

➤ **Predatory aggression:** triggered by the presence of a natural quarry.

➤ **Antipredatory aggression:** caused by the presence of a predator.

➤ **Territorial aggression:** in defence of a cat's domain against an intruder.

➤ **Dominant aggression:** in response to a challenge to the individual or because it wants to gain access to a critical resource.

➤ **Maternal aggression:** this is brought about by the proximity of any agent that represents a threat to a mother's litter.

➤ **Weaning aggression:** caused by the growing independence of the offspring; the parents threaten or even gently attack their young.

➤ **Disciplined parental aggression:** this is provoked by various stimuli such as out-of-hours breastfeeding, rough or excessively long games, distancing, and similar actions.

➤ **Sexual aggression:** triggered by female cats that wish to mate or establish a more long-lasting union.

➤ **Sex-related aggression:** prompted by the same stimuli that trigger sexual behaviours.

➤ **Intermale aggression:** stimulated by the presence of another male competitor.

➤ **Fear aggression:** due to confinement or feeling cornered and unable to escape, or the presence of a threatening agent.

➤ **Irritable aggression:** provoked by the presence of any assailable living creature or object.

➤ **Instrumental aggression:** any change in the environment, as a result of any of the aggressive conducts described already, that increases the likelihood of an aggressive behaviour occurring in similar situations.

MODIFIED MOYER'S CLASSIFICATION

- ➤ **Dominance aggression.**
- ➤ **Intrasexual aggression** (both between males and between females).
- ➤ **Predatory aggression.**
- ➤ **Pain aggression.**
- ➤ **Instrumental aggression.**
- ➤ **Fear aggression.**
- ➤ **Territorial aggression.**
- ➤ **Maternal aggression.**
- ➤ **Redirected aggression.**
- ➤ **Aggression secondary to pathophysiological changes.**

SOCIOPATHIES

Other authors with an alternative approach to animal behaviour do not define aggression problems according to a strict classification, instead they discuss sociopathies and differentiate between two states:

- ➤ Reactive sociopathy: characterised by a regulated and organised sequence of aggression which the authors consider a perfectly normal social behaviour for cats.
- ➤ Instrumentalised sociopathy (secondary hyperaggressive): evidenced by the loss of aggression-regulating elements, considered an absolute disease state.

These investigators also indicate that hierarchical, irritable, and territorial aggression behaviours make up the hallmark trident of clinical signs observed in sociopathies.

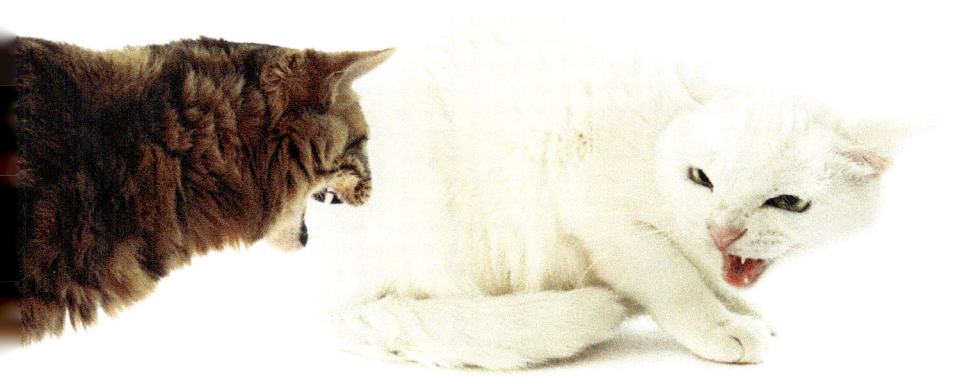

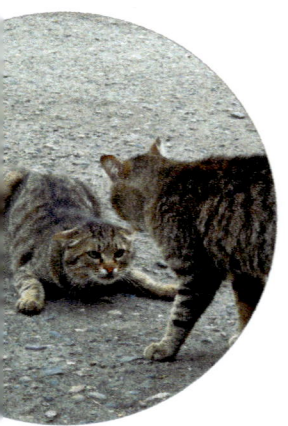

INTRASEXUAL AGGRESSION

This is the most common form of aggression displayed by male cats. Testosterone is the impetus for this behaviour; it stimulates masculinisation of the male brain even before birth.

In adult males, testosterone has a selective action on the portion of the brain that regulates aggressive behaviour. It also causes the skin on the neck of male cats to thicken.

Males not only fight so they can mate with females, but also for territories and social rank (higher ranked animals have preferential access to critical resources) (Fig. 3). While castration corrects this behaviour effectively in 90 % of these cases, in practice, the owner needs to appreciate that the cat will still try to escape at night, as socialising in neighbourhood gatherings is not regulated by testosterone. Castration will, however, reduce the frequency and ferocity with which male cats fight.

Progestogen therapy using appropriate doses of medroxyprogesterone acetate or megestrol acetate is effective in both cats whose owners do not opt for castration and the 10 % of castrated male cats that still continue to fight. It is important that owners respect their cat's circadian rhythm by administering these hormone therapies late in the evening. Veterinary surgeons should advise owners to confine their cat to a suitable location while receiving the treatment, make them aware of the possible side effects of this type of hormone therapy, and, if feasible, perform blood tests before and after progestogen administration.

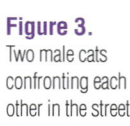

Figure 3.
Two male cats confronting each other in the street.

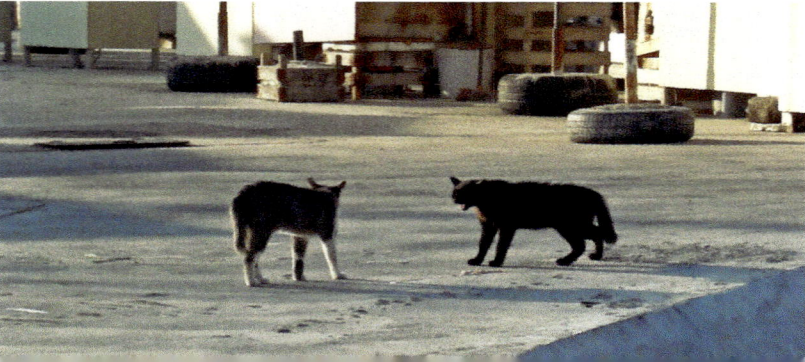

> In the case of intrasexual aggression between females (much less frequent), hormone therapy is not an option and surgical castration is ineffective; therefore, the only choices are behavioural therapy or physical separation of the warring animals.

TREATMENT

➤ **Behavioural therapy:** remote correction of conducts displayed by aggressive individuals (in applicable cases).

➤ **Surgical treatment:** castration.

➤ **Drug treatment:** choice of medication within the indicated therapeutic range:

  ➤ Buspirone: 1–5 mg/cat/day, split over two doses, orally.

  ➤ Fluoxetine: 0.5–1.0 mg/kg, every 24 h, orally.

  ➤ Megestrol acetate: 2.5–10.0 mg/cat, every 24 h, orally. Reduce the initial dose progressively.

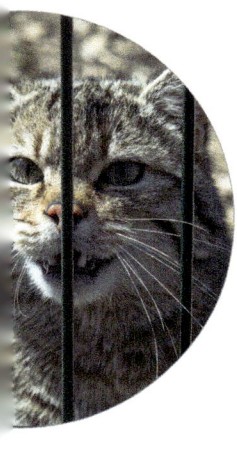

TERRITORIAL AGGRESSION

Both males and females, whether castrated or entire, will defend their territories regardless of their hormonal status. This is a normal conduct that only becomes problematic when there are two or more cats living together in the same household. For males, progestogen therapy is helpful for the first 2–3 weeks while the new housemates develop a level of mutual tolerance. Antianxiety therapy may also prove effective; for example, the use of benzodiazepines (whilst always paying attention to their potential side effects). Personally, I prefer to administer azapirones (buspirone) or serotonin reuptake inhibitors (fluoxetine, paroxetine, etc.) rather than benzodiazepine.

The solution to this type of behavioural alteration will obviously depend on the degree of overcrowding and the method the owner applies to manage the situation.

TREATMENT

➤ **Behavioural therapy:** remote correction of conducts displayed by aggressive individuals (in applicable cases).

➤ **Surgical treatment:** castration (males).

➤ **Drug treatment:** choice of medication within the indicated therapeutic range:

  ➤ Buspirone: 1–5 mg/cat/day, split over two doses, orally.
  ➤ Fluoxetine: 0.5–1.0 mg/kg, every 24 h, orally.
  ➤ Megestrol acetate: 2.5–10.0 mg/cat, every 24 h, orally. Reduce the initial dose progressively.

PREDATORY AGGRESSION DIRECTED TOWARDS PEOPLE

Hunting comprises two behavioural components – play and aggression. A deviation from this normal behaviour is whenever the cat attacks the ankles of people walking by. While it is never a dangerous act of aggression and is more like a game, it still represents a nuisance or even frightens some owners (Fig. 4). As the animal is chasing an escaping prey, the solution is to stop when you feel the attack and discourage the cat from persisting with the conduct. In more severe cases, where a very sensitive and fearful owner is involved, the best advice is to correct the behaviour using a water pistol or compressed air spray.

Aggression directed towards people is not strictly speaking a behavioural disorder, rather it is a consequence secondary to other behavioural alterations such as pain aggression, redirected aggression, and so on. In fact, when living with a human family, cats develop and exhibit the same behaviours towards the people in their social group as they do towards other cats, this includes both pleasant (playing, affection) and unpleasant conducts (aggression).

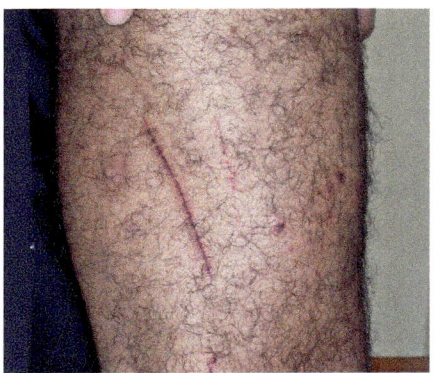 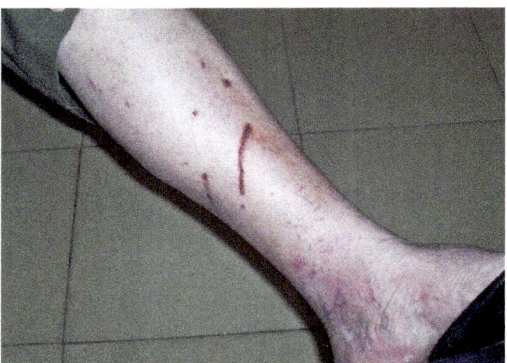

Figure 4. Injuries caused by a cat's predatory aggression towards people.

> House cats belong to an asocial species, so familiarity with and respect for their specific behavioural patterns will facilitate pleasant coexistence between owners and their cats.

If vets can make owners understand and accept that giving their cats a certain degree of freedom of choice will avert major conflicts, they will have acted professionally and prevented a lot of future problems.

Water pistols or compressed air sprays are a very effective and simple means of eliminating attacks on people.

TREATMENT

Drug treatment is particularly helpful and often an essential resource to resolve the problem.

In general, cats displaying predatory aggression towards people should be given serotonin reuptake inhibitors; fluoxetine has proven to be the most effective in cats. The azapirones paroxetine and buspirone are also viable options at dosages of 1–5 mg/cat/day split over two doses. They regulate serotonin and are known to be very effective in cats. These drugs must be administered for at least 5 weeks, but also for the shortest period possible because they can produce unwanted side effects.

Anticonvulsants, sedatives, and tranquillisers, while their use is described and indicated in the literature, should be used with caution as some of them can trigger a paradoxical effect in cats.

➤ Buspirone: 1–5 mg/cat/day, split over two doses, orally.
➤ Fluoxetine: 0.5–1.0 mg/kg, every 24 h, orally.

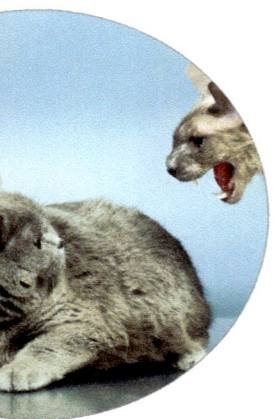

REDIRECTED AGGRESSION, OR AGGRESSION LEARNED THROUGH FEAR OR PAIN

Redirected aggression, or aggression learned through fear or pain, is another form of aggression towards people. When a cat cannot attack its target, it gets frustrated and attacks the nearest thing in its vicinity, usually the owner who often approaches to stroke their pet given its agitated behaviour.

A classic example is that of a cat looking out of the window at another cat in the street. The cat becomes restless and frustrated because it cannot chase the other cat off its turf, as it is trapped inside, so it redirects its pent-up aggression onto whoever approaches to pet it. This situation can evolve into learned aggression if it is not dealt with and controlled in time.

If a cat attacks or threatens another cat, a dog, or a person and gains some sort of benefit, it is very likely to repeat this behaviour. For instance, if a child pulls a cat's tail which then retaliates by scratching, the child will leave the cat alone and maybe avoid it altogether in the future; the cat has learnt that scratching or attacking the child has a positive outcome, so it will do it again, even when the child is not bothering it. The cat may also generalise the conduct to attacking all the people living in the house. Treatment involves direct action to correct the behaviour using a water sprayer or compressed air spray each time the cat displays the aggression, combined with rewards for nonviolent behaviour. Besides being professionally unethical, direct physical punishment is totally contraindicated in cats because it creates a negative relationship between the animal and the person punishing it and causes more behavioural problems than it resolves.

Cats normally avoid confrontation with anyone or any animals that frighten them, so dangerous situations arise when they are left without an escape route. Pain and fear are very strong and significant stimuli in terms of unleashing feline aggression. This kind of aggression is the main reason behind children receiving bites or scratches. The best means of approaching the situation is undoubtedly for the owner to treat the animal correctly and control the children in the house.

Cats will almost always react aggressively when undergoing painful medical procedures unless they have received a correct upbringing, appropriate handling from their owner, and developed trust in their owner. When a cat exhibits aggression and requires a medical intervention, veterinary surgeons can use (for cats inside a carrier) a mixture of acepromazine (0.2 mL) and ketamine hydrochloride (0.3 mL) administered orally by using a syringe to fire the solution into the patient's mouth when open during an aggressive gesture. The medication will immobilise the cat for a few minutes giving the veterinary professional time to complete some procedures such as curing a wound or administering an intramuscular anaesthesia.

TREATMENT

Treatment consists of avoiding the frustrating situation that triggers the attack. If the situation has already established itself, the conduct should be deflected by enticing the cat to practice a different activity from that which stimulates the aggression (continuing with the first example, the aim would be to divert the cat's attention to an activity other than looking out the window). In the severest of cases, the negative behaviour can be corrected using a water pistol or air spray device. Depending on the severity of the situation, psychoactive drugs may be indicated:

➤ Buspirone: 1–5 mg/cat/day, split over two doses, orally.
➤ Fluoxetine: 0.5–1.0 mg/kg, every 24 h, orally.

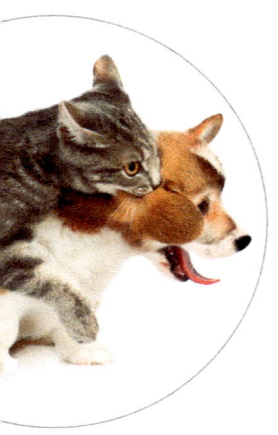

FELINE SOCIAL AGGRESSION

This corresponds to aggression from an adult cat towards a kitten or young cat that has recently joined the household. This behaviour occurs because cats sometimes perceive other individuals as if they belonged to another species depending on the other cat's developmental stage. Young cats display a sociable behavioural pattern until the age of 8–12 months, at which point they achieve independence and adopt the typical asocial behaviour characteristic of adult males. As such, when a kitten approaches an adult cat to indulge its gregarious behaviour, the adult may attack and seriously injure the kitten. This problem can be overcome by introducing two young cats into the house at the same time. However, owners do not usually consider this option, so they must be made to understand that they cannot leave an older and younger cat together without supervision and it is the owner who must fulfil the role of the kitten's playmate.

After a few weeks the adult cat normally comes to accept the new kitten and the problem dissipates completely when the latter is 8–9 months old, since both cats now follow the same behavioural pattern.

Adult cats may also direct this sort of aggression towards other newly arrived, nonfeline housemates.

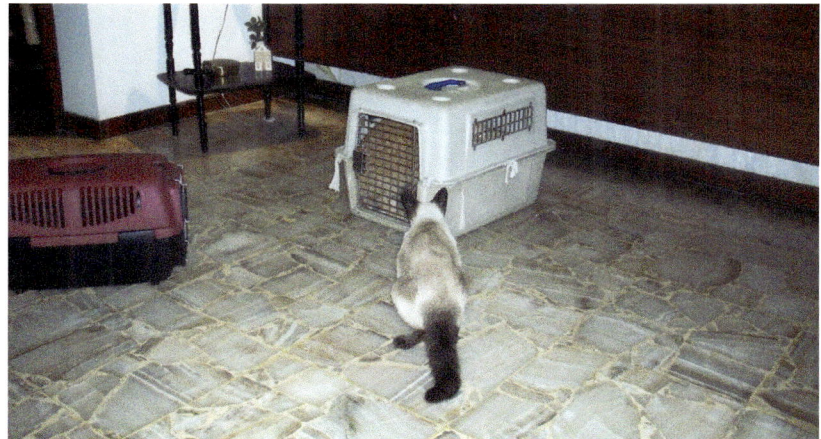

Figure 5. An adult cat getting used to the presence of a kitten (inside the carrier).

TREATMENT

➤ **Behavioural therapy:** start by placing the kitten in a carrier, thus allowing the adult to get used to the young cat's presence while also ensuring its safety (Fig. 5).

➤ **Drug treatment:** drugs are of limited use, but in certain cases the resident adult can be medicated if the arrival of a new kitten results in an excessively stressful situation that triggers agitated behaviour. Selective serotonin reuptake inhibitors or azapirones can be administered in such cases:

  ➤ Buspirone: 1–5 mg/cat/day, split over two doses, orally.
  ➤ Fluoxetine: 0.5–1.0 mg/kg, every 24 h, orally.

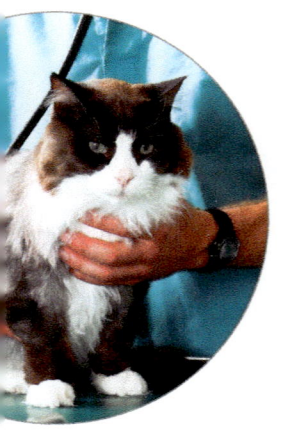

AGGRESSION DUE TO PATHOPHYSIOLOGICAL CONDITIONS

Thyroid disorders can trigger alterations in the aggression patterns normally displayed by cats (as they also do in other species). This is why vets must first attempt to identify or rule out any underlying diseases before assessing and diagnosing the patient's behavioural problem.

Epilepsy is another clinical condition that is sometimes associated with aggressive conducts. In fact, abnormally aggressive behaviour is a common sign of subclinical epileptic seizures.

Besides, any pathophysiological condition that is a cause of malaise for the animal is a potential source of an overly aggressive response.

Changes in personality have been reported in cats that have received a prolonged general anaesthesia with barbiturates or ketamine, possibly because they suffered a lengthy period of neuronal anoxia.

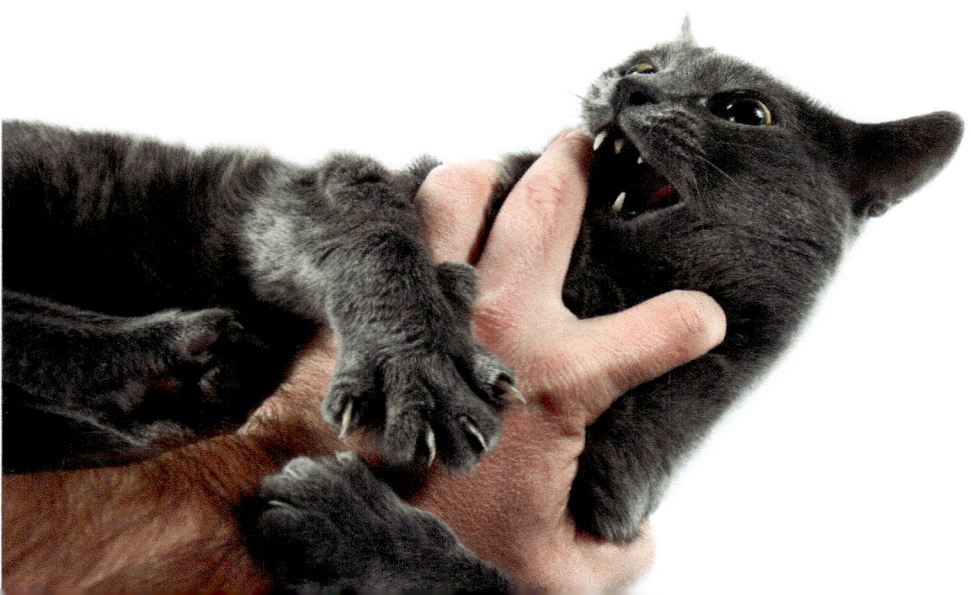

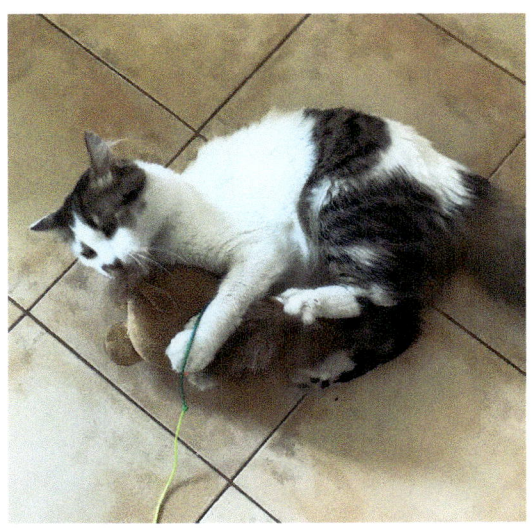

Figure 6. A cat biting and clasping onto a toy that it has just captured.

TREATMENT

The treatment of this class of behavioural disorders involves the correct diagnosis of the underlying clinical disease responsible for the behavioural problem. However, once the clinical condition has been resolved, the animal often continues to exhibit the anomalous conduct. If this occurs, the drugs mentioned earlier and behavioural therapy adapted to the patient's problem may both prove useful.

Irrespective of the type of aggression disorder observed in a house cat, one therapeutic technique always turns out to be helpful; channelling the animal's aggression, without focusing on the inherent cause, through predatory games with the owner. The owner just needs a piece of string, a soft toy, and their own goodwill. Tie a metre-long piece of string around the soft toy and entice the cat to stalk and catch it. When it captures the toy, let go so the cat can play with it. The size of the toy should allow the cat to clutch it with its front paws and strike it with its rear paws whilst biting (Fig. 6).

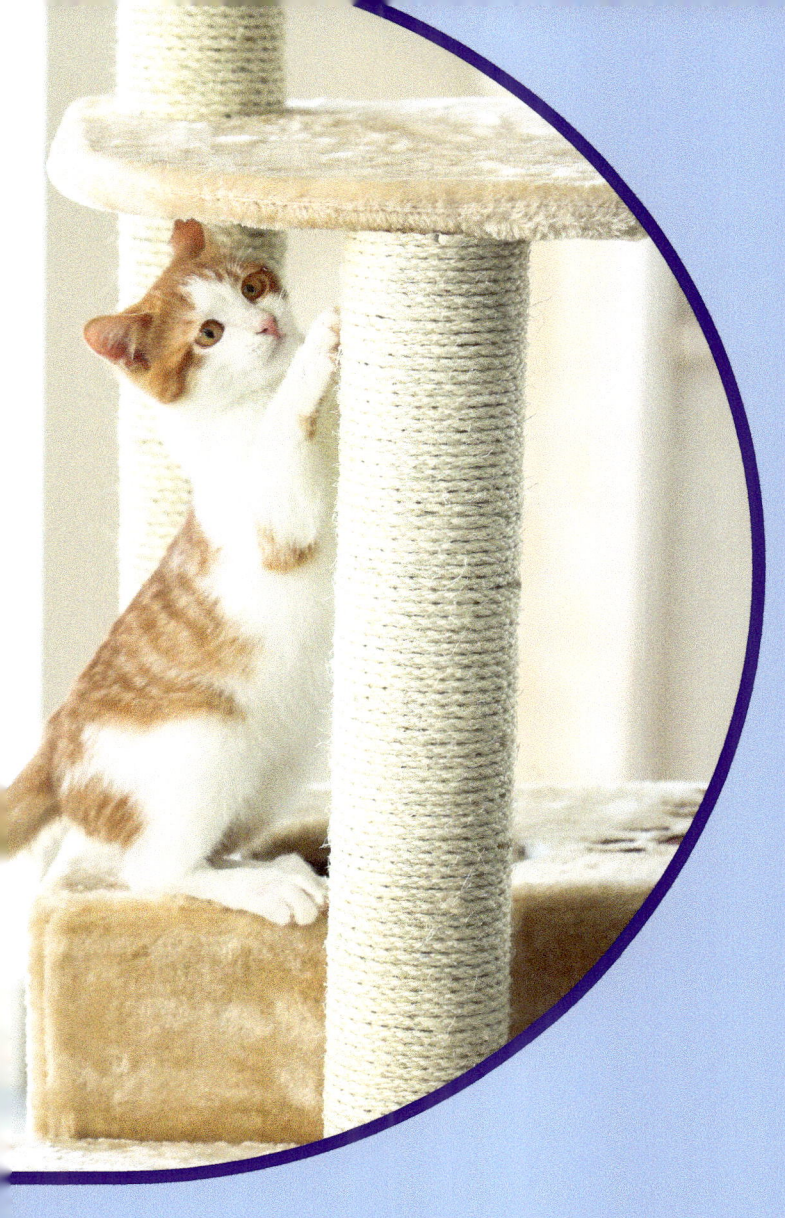

DISORDERS ASSOCIATED WITH ENVIRONMENTAL STRESS CAT STEREOTYPIES

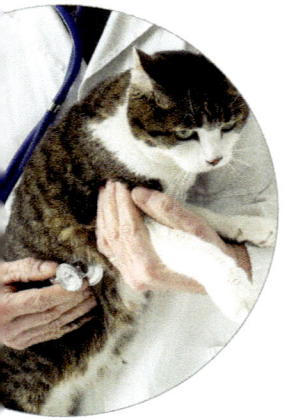

INTRODUCTION

Stereotyped behaviour or compulsive disorder is one of the most frequently encountered behavioural alterations observed in cats and dogs during day-to-day clinical practice. Due to its complex and multifactorial origin, it is also one of the most regularly misdiagnosed conditions as it is more often associated with dermatological, neurological, or hormonal diseases rather than behavioural alterations.

A stereotyped behaviour, or stereotypy, is a constant, repetitive action with no apparent objective in the context in which it is exhibited. This definition is not strictly accurate, as stereotypies have different degrees of variation. Some are not actually repetitive, while others are repetitive but include a clear objective (e.g. tail chasing). Animals that display this behaviour are often suffering from stress due to an impoverished environment.

> Stereotyped behaviours are abnormal expressions of normal behaviours typically observed in the species, for example, grooming, vocalisation, locomotion, etc.

It is important to take into account that an animal's compulsive behaviours are, in many cases, a response to the high levels of anxiety it is suffering as a result of frustration or confusion caused by its environmental living conditions.

As with all behaviours, stereotypies are influenced by both environmental and genetic components; in other words, some breeds have a greater predisposition than others to develop this type of disorder in certain environmental conditions.

The most widely recognised stereotyped behaviours in cats are wool sucking, tail chasing, tail mutilation, excessive grooming, psychogenic dermatitis, and feline hyperaesthesia syndrome.

Learning about the causes of the stereotypies (Box 1) can help improve our understanding of this disorder.

Box 1. Origin of different stereotypies.

Pathophysiological causes	Genetic	➤ **Physical:** inherited abnormalities such as deafness, hydrocephalus, and so on, that lead to behavioural disorders. ➤ **Behavioural:** inherited behavioural disorders such as narcolepsy, wool sucking, etc.
	Acquired	➤ Conditions such as neurological and infectious diseases (rabies, etc.), malnutrition, intoxication, and so on, that leave physical sequelae and in turn cause behavioural alterations.
Experiential causes	Developmental	➤ Behaviours arising from experiences endured by the animal during a critical stage of its behavioural development, for example, poor socialisation.
	Reactive	➤ Behaviours the animal develops in response to its living conditions; for example, mistreatment, an impoverished environment, and a lack of exercise, amongst others.
	Conditioned	➤ Behaviours resulting from animal conditioning, generally because the owner reinforces the behaviour; for example, the owner encourages tail chasing because they think it is a game.

When the animal faces a situation of conflict or frustration that produces a high degree of stress or anxiety, it will try to cope through different behaviours (which always derive from species-specific behaviours). These behaviours could be:

➤ Redirected behaviour: normal behaviour directed towards a subject other than that which generates the triggering stimulus.
➤ Displacement behaviour: normal behaviour but at the wrong time; for example, grooming, vocalisation, etc.
➤ Neurotic behaviour: abnormal behaviour that does not stem from a normal conduct such as self-mutilation, tail chasing, and so on.
➤ Stereotyped behaviour*: constant, repetitive behaviour with no apparent purpose and which stems from a displacement activity.
➤ Compulsive behaviour*: the animal loses control of when it starts and finishes the stereotypy.
➤ Vacuum activity*: normal behaviour directed towards a nonexistent subject; for example, licking the air, chasing nonexistent flies, etc.

* Displacement activities

PATHOPHYSIOLOGY

When we integrate all the concepts discussed previously, we can conclude that it is hard to delimit the aetiology and pathophysiology of compulsive syndromes because in practice the origin and development of a stereotyped behaviour are inseparable.

When a cat is confronted by a conflict or environmental stress it will try to deal with the situation through a displacement activity whose genetic basis is founded on normal species-specific behaviours, but which could develop into a stereotypy depending on the animal's life experiences, its environment-induced frustration, the intensity of the stress-inducing stimulus, and its owner's response.

From a physiological perspective, this conduct is preserved in the specific neuropathological changes due to the alterations in the brain biochemistry of animals exhibiting these behaviours.

Stereotypies are induced by stimulants of the dopamine system (amphetamines, apomorphine), stress due to anxiety, and owner reinforcement of the animal's conduct.

We also known that stereotyped behaviours are maintained by endogenous opioids, released in stressful situations, which activate dopaminergic neurons.

In many cases, subclinical temporal lobe epilepsy has been confirmed as the cause of some stereotypies.

In practice, a lack of adequate interaction with other cats and animals or people, mainly during the socialisation period spanning from 3–9 weeks, may predispose the animal to exhibit stereotypies as an adult, even though it lives in a suitable environment.

So, compulsive behaviours in cats can be simultaneously placed in several categories of abnormal behaviour.

> Stereotypies are the manifestation of an animal's previous or current conflict with its environment, its early life experiences, and its genetic predisposition (e.g. wool sucking in oriental breeds).

CLINICAL SIGNS

Some anomalous conducts can derive from a normal movement pattern and transform into stereotypies or compulsive behaviours, these also involve neurosis and by definition are not species-specific behaviours. Accordingly, the clinical signs of stereotypies based on normal patterns can be found in Table 1.

Table 1. Clinical signs of stereotypies based on normal movement patterns.

Pattern	Clinical signs of the stereotypy
Grooming	➤ Compulsive self-licking ➤ Hair chewing ➤ Acral granuloma (a cutaneous lump as a result of inflammation caused by incessant licking)
Diet	➤ Polydipsia ➤ Polyphagia ➤ Wool sucking ➤ Excessive drooling ➤ Fabric eating
Locomotion	➤ Sudden movements of the body ➤ Running and jumping ➤ Freezing of gait ➤ Shaking or nodding the head
Vocalisation	➤ Constant meowing ➤ Constant crying ➤ Self-mutilation with or without vocalisation
Neurosis	➤ Regular aggression directed at people ➤ Teeth chattering ➤ Hunting nonexistent prey ➤ Staring into space

In addition to these clinical signs, any other signs noted during the anamnesis that are of a repetitive nature, harmful to the animal, or which the patient cannot control in terms of when they start and end should also be recorded.

MOST COMMON CAT STEREOTYPIES

The diseases most frequently encountered in the context of a compulsive syndrome or stereotyped behaviour in cats are:
- Excessive grooming: feline psychogenic alopecia.
- Feline hyperaesthesia.
- Wool sucking.
- Tail chasing, with or without self-mutilation.

DIAGNOSIS

The diagnosis revolves around the following points:
- Data gathered during the anamnesis in an attempt to identify the cause: onset of the condition, context in which the animal exhibits the behaviour, etc.
- Identification of the origin: primarily genetic or environmental.
- Direct observation of the patient's behaviour, the owner–patient relationship, and their living environment, as well as an understanding of any frustration-inducing factors. Additionally, the veterinary surgeon should observe if the animal displays other, nonstereotyped behavioural alterations.

Organic causes must be ruled out through complementary methods (analysis of hormone levels, an electroencephalogram, allergy testing, X-rays, etc.) and a probable environmental cause should be established.

In the case of stereotypies with associated dermatological diseases of uncertain origin, corticosteroids can be used as a means of diagnosis.

It would be entirely incorrect to diagnose "boredom" as the cause of the problem, although it may form part of the cause.

> Diagnosis is based on the clinical signs and information collected during the anamnesis, always provided that any clinical conditions are ruled out.

TREATMENT

Treatment is based on establishing a combination of behavioural therapy, adjusting the animal's environment, and drug treatment.

BEHAVIOURAL THERAPY

Behavioural therapy consists of:

➤ **Counterconditioning**: this involves teaching the animal a behaviour that is incompatible with the stereotypy.

➤ **Distraction from the behaviour**: attracting the animal's attention when it is engrossed in the stereotypy using noises, food, toys, and so on.

➤ **Systematic desensitisation**: entails progressively introducing the stimulus that triggers the stereotypy, the aim being to gradually cause the animal less anxiety.

➤ **Aversion therapy**: this is a behavioural modification technique through which the cat associates its behaviour with an unpleasant consequence (e.g. using devices that expel compressed air and make a sound, by applying bitter substances to the site where the animal compulsively licks itself, etc.).

MODIFICATION OF THE PATIENT'S ENVIRONMENT

The first step is to clearly identify the triggering stimulus of the stereotypy, so it may be withdrawn before changing the animal's routine.

INTERACTION WITH THE OWNER

Many owners either directly punish or hug and stroke their cats when they exhibit the compulsive behaviour, which only serves to reinforce the stereotypy. Therefore, it is very important to instruct the owner to ignore the animal's behaviour and distract the animal with a game; they should never exert a direct punishment. It is essential that the owner changes the way they deal with their pet if they are interacting incorrectly.

CAT PHEROMONES

Cat pheromones are very useful in the treatment of all behavioural disorders in cats, but particularly in those related to an impoverished environment, stress, or anxiety. They can generate a feeling of wellbeing and calm in cats. The most effective devices are ambient diffusers. They release pheromones for approximately 1 month when plugged into an electrical wall socket. Only cats can smell feline pheromones – they are harmless and odourless for people and other animals.

ENVIRONMENTAL ENRICHMENT

This approach aims to provide indoor cats with a stimulating and enriched environment that improves their lives. There is a range of options, as such the owner should be encouraged to consider different alternatives to enrich their cat's environment, depending on their lifestyle and type of home.

Enclosures that allow the animal to safely access outdoor areas make a great resource (Fig. 1). If outdoor access is limited or unavailable, owners must improve their pet's indoor environment by providing entertainment and stimulation (Fig. 2).

In homes where several cats live together, they can be kept in cages from an early age to help define each cat's individual territory. Kittens should be familiarised with the setting by placing them in a cage large enough to cover all their needs (food, water, litter box, and sleeping area). They can also include toys or areas for climbing and hiding. When the owner is available to interact, the kitten should be let out of its cage to explore and play throughout the house and interact with the owner. Over time, the cage can be left open for increasingly longer periods until it remains open permanently, allowing the animal free access. As all of the cat's needs can be

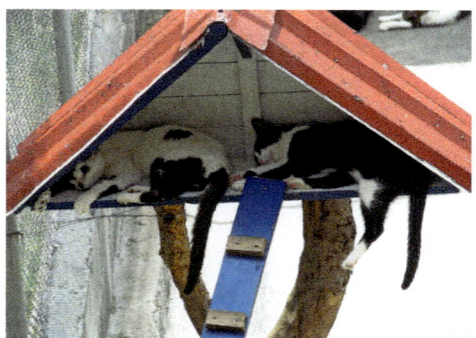

Figure 1. The use of enclosures will allow cats to access outdoor areas.

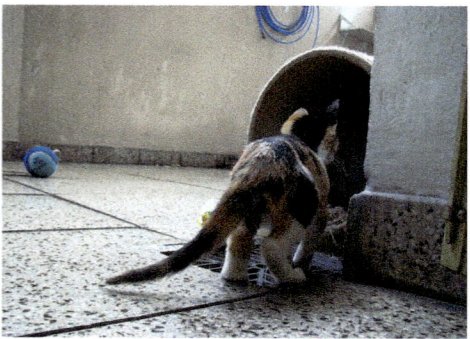

Figure 2. The indoor environment should be improved to provide the cat with entertainment and stimulation.

fulfilled within the cage, it will regard the small area as its own territory.

Areas for climbing (Fig. 3) and relaxing on shelves (Fig. 4) also offer exercise and security, as they help maintain social order. Commercially available cat trees and furniture provide several areas for climbing and hiding (Fig. 5), as well as individual platforms; they also offer extra benefits when placed close to a window (Fig. 6). When the owner does not have time to interact with the cat, they can use devices or toys that entertain the animal, for example, feathers hung in different locations. Environmental enrichment can sometimes include the acquisition of another animal. Obviously, each case requires a personalised study of the environmental conditions (owner's lifestyle, cat's habitat, time available, etc.).

Taking into account the owner's lifestyle, the veterinary professional should advise them on how to optimise their pet's health and wellbeing. Lifestyle, environment, and diet should all be discussed during the first consultation. If the cat is given processed foods, they can be hidden in different locations to simulate hunting and gathering. This will entertain the cat and limit its intake better than a tray full of food.

DRUG TREATMENT

Stereotypies can be induced by drugs that activate the dopamine system (amphetamine and apomorphine); furthermore, endogenous opioid peptides released by the brain in stressful situations activate dopaminergic neurons, which means stereotyped behaviours respond favourably to opioid receptor blockers and dopamine antagonists.

Haloperidol inhibits stereotypies induced experimentally in cats with dopamine and dextroamphetamine.

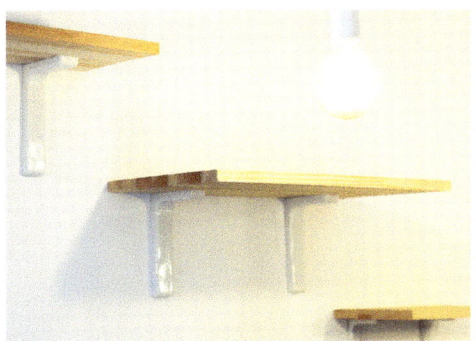

Figure 3. Climbing area.

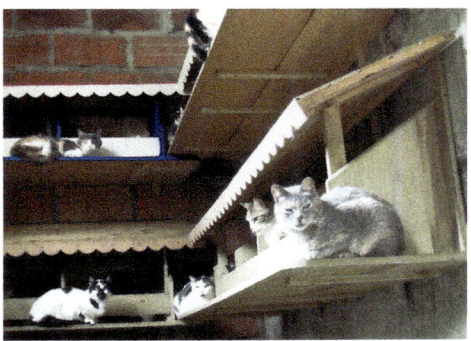

Figure 4. Wall shelving.

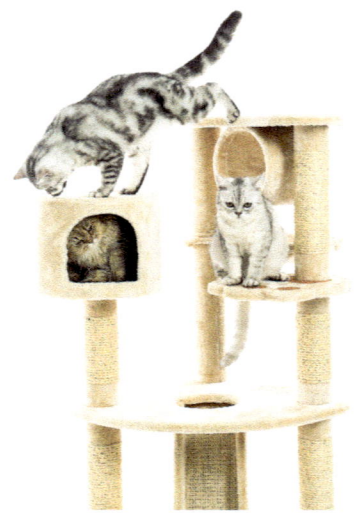

Figure 5. Cat furniture with climbing and hiding areas.

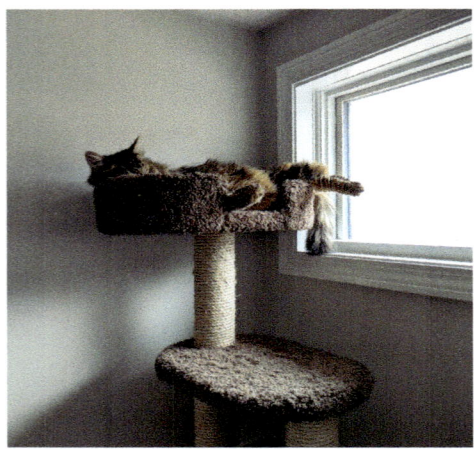

Figure 6. Cat furniture placed next to a window.

SEROTONIN REUPTAKE INHIBITORS

Stereotypies are generally treated with serotonin reuptake inhibitors as the first-line drug: fluoxetine, at a dose of 0.5–1.0 mg/kg/day, is the most effective, paroxetine is another option.

These drugs have some unwanted side effects such as gastrointestinal complaints (including anorexia and diarrhoea, although these can be mitigated by starting at a low dose and increasing up to the therapeutic dose), agitation, and insomnia.

> Selective serotonin reuptake inhibitors have significantly milder side effects than those associated with tricyclic antidepressants and are much less unpredictable than the potential adverse effects of benzodiazepines.

TRICYCLIC ANTIDEPRESSANTS

The second most popular group of drugs are tricyclic antidepressants such as clomipramine (0.5–1.5 mg/day, orally), imipramine (2.2–4.4 mg/kg/day), and amitriptyline (5–10 mg/day in two oral doses).

These drugs must be administered for at least 5 weeks and then for the least time possible thereafter because they all produce adverse side effects, including:

➤ Cardiovascular effects: orthostatic hypotension, decreased cardiac conduction, and antiarrhythmic properties. These do not represent a significant problem in healthy animals, but vets should exercise utmost precaution when administering them to patients with partial heart block, as they may suffer complete heart block.

➤ Anticholinergic effects: these are the most common side effects, resulting from a block in muscarinic receptor activity. They include mydriasis, dry mouth, urinary retention, and constipation.

➤ Antihistamine effects.

➤ Sedative effects.

ANTICONVULSANTS

Anticonvulsants have a therapeutic purpose if the origin of the stereotypy was accurately diagnosed as subclinical epilepsy.

ANXIOLYTICS

In most cases, patients with a stereotypy also exhibit a high degree of anxiety, so they are treated with anxiolytic agents. Benzodiazepines are the first-line anxiolytics, particularly clonazepam at a dose of 0.5–2.2 mg/cat/day given orally, as its administration is more practical for the owner and it can be given in 1 or 2 daily doses, depending on each case.

The main disadvantage of benzodiazepines is the potential for addiction, so they must be discontinued gradually. There have been a few reports of idiopathic hepatic necrosis associated with the oral use of benzodiazepines, mainly diazepam. Additionally, administration of this drug group can reduce the effectiveness of behaviour modification techniques because they cause amnesia and therefore interfere with the patient's learning capacity. Special attention must be paid when using diazepam in cats as it can occasionally produce a paradoxical effect.

Buspirone is also indicated for cats; it is a nonbenzodiazepine anxiolytic from the azapirone group. It modulates serotonin, by acting on pre- and postsynaptic serotonin 1A receptors, has practically no side effects, and can be discontinued abruptly, unlike benzodiazepine derivatives. However, buspirone does not have such a potent therapeutic action as the aforementioned drugs, but it has given good results when combined with behaviour modification techniques and can be used safely in cats. Cats should be administered 2.5–5.0 mg/cat/day, spread across two doses.

> It is totally contraindicated to punish the animal when it exhibits the stereotypy or stop it from carrying out the action.

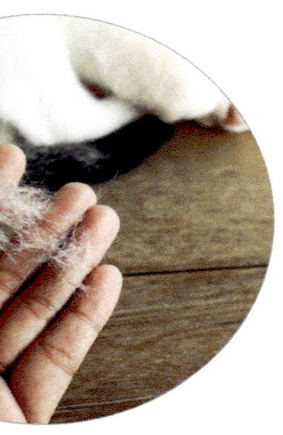

EXCESSIVE GROOMING (FELINE PSYCHOGENIC ALOPECIA)

This is basically a compulsive licking disorder.

ANAMNESIS

It is important to observe and record the following data during the anamnesis:

➤ Significant environmental changes: try to establish a link between any environmental changes and the onset of the problem (moving to a new house, birth of a baby, arrival of a new animal, death of a family member, etc.).

➤ The animal's behaviour (at home or in the clinic): it is vital to identify when the cat exhibits the licking behaviour (if it does it in other environments, only in the presence of a certain member of the household, when it does not receive attention, etc.).

➤ Other behavioural changes: aggressiveness, unruliness, urine marking behaviour, etc.

➤ The owner–pet relationship: if they have a good relationship or the cat tries to escape from the owner (which could be a sign that the owner punishes or scolds the animal, which in turn may aggravate the condition).

➤ Characteristics of the alopecic area: if the hair loss coincides with the areas the cat can reach with its tongue (Figs. 7 and 8), the alopecia is greater on one side of the body than the other (Fig. 9), etc. This observation should be complemented with a microscopic examination of the patient's hair (trichogram). This will reveal whether or not the loose hairs have capillary bulbs, so you can differentiate between hair loss due to internal causes (e.g. hormonal) or because of the licking (in which case there will be no capillary bulb).

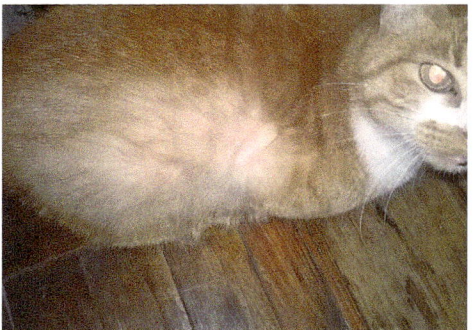

Figure 7. Feline psychogenic alopecia. The hair loss affects the zones the cat can reach with its tongue.

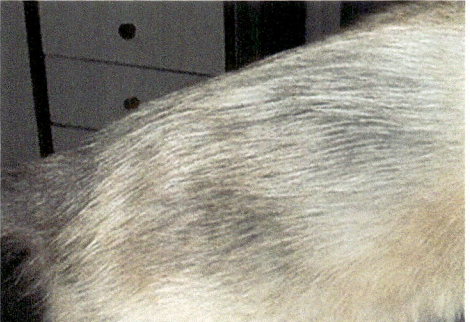

Figure 8. Feline psychogenic alopecia. The hair removal affects the zones the cat can reach with its tongue.

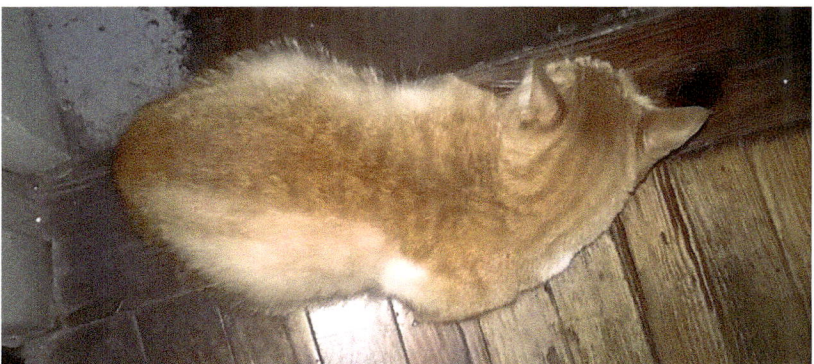

Figure 9. There is more hair loss on one side of the body than the other.

BEHAVIOURAL DISORDERS IN CATS

DIAGNOSIS

Diagnosis is based on:

➤ Information recorded during the anamnesis.

➤ Trichogram: in the case of feline psychogenic alopecia, hair taken from the area of interest will appear broken and lack the bulb. Although this characteristic is not pathognomonic, it does help with the diagnosis, as hairs are not broken in hormonal alopecia and they still possess the bulb.

➤ Exclusion of any underlying medical problems: such as dermatitis of different origins and diseases that produce pruritus, in which case corticosteroids are occasionally used to make a diagnosis of exclusion. In the case of dermatological conditions (flea allergy dermatitis, atopic dermatitis, etc.), a triamcinolone acetate injection (0.11–0.22 mg/kg, subcutaneously or intramuscularly) can be administered if there is any doubt about the origin of the problem and the patient reassessed 1 week later. Corticosteroids will not resolve the compulsive behaviour, but they will address the aforementioned conditions. Again, this is not a pathognomonic trait, but it helps considerably in the diagnosis.

TREATMENT

➤ **Behavioural therapy**: desensitisation and distraction from the behaviour.

➤ **Environment modification**: elimination of the stressful cause, environment enrichment, appropriate management by the animal's owner, and so on.

➤ **Drug treatment** within the indicated therapeutic range.
  ➤ Clonazepam*: 0.25–1.10 mg/cat, every 12 h, orally.
  ➤ Buspirone*: 1–5 mg/cat/day, split over two doses, orally.
  ➤ Fluoxetine*: 0.5–1.0 mg/kg, every 24 h, orally.
  ➤ Diazepam: 0.5–2.0 mg/cat, every 8 h, orally.
  ➤ Amitriptyline: 2.5–5.0 mg/cat, every 12 h, orally.
  ➤ Clomipramine: 0.5–1.5 mg/cat, every 24 h, orally.
  ➤ Megestrol acetate: 2.5–10.0 mg/cat, every 24 h, orally, and progressively decrease the initial dose.
  ➤ Prednisone: 1–2 mg/kg, every 48 h. orally, for 10 days.

* The author's preferred drugs, but they are not the only viable options available.

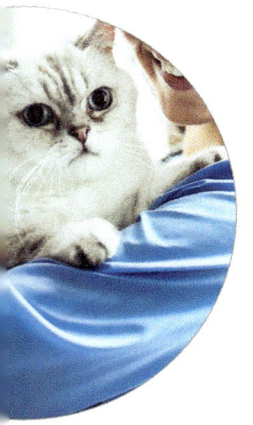

FELINE HYPERAESTHESIA

ANAMNESIS

It is important to observe and record the following data during the anamnesis:

➤ Significant environmental changes that coincided with the onset of the problematic behaviour; as with all these disorders, the vet must seek a correlation between an environmental change and the onset of the issue. The signs may appear spontaneously or intermittently.

➤ The animal's behaviour: the main observable signs are dilated pupils, vocalisation, muscle spasms, sudden terror with or without associated defaecation, aggression towards people, etc. The clinical manifestations vary widely from one cat to another. The most notable conduct is the cat's exaggerated response when touched in the dorsal region. In fact, often they do not even need to be touched as they exhibit the action spontaneously: the skin in the area contracts and wrinkles, the animal vocalises, arches its back, becomes frightened and excited, and compulsively scratches its back.

➤ Other behavioural changes: the observation of changes in marking behaviour, aggressiveness, or fearful behaviour can indicate the animal's predisposition to behavioural changes, as these conducts can be confused with dermatological conditions.

➤ The affected area: hyper-reactivity when touched in the dorso-lumbar area. Observation of self-inflicted lesions, whether due to scratching or over-zealous licking (Fig. 10).

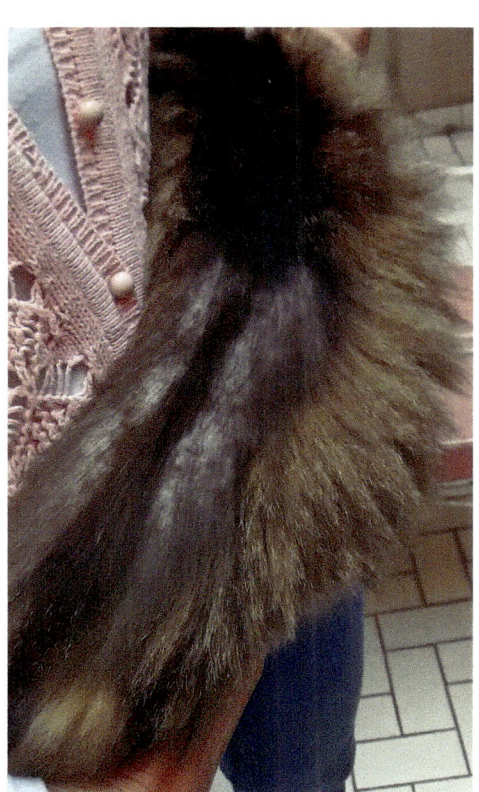

Figure 10. Patient with feline hyperaesthesia.

DIAGNOSIS

Diagnosis is based on:

➤ Data collected during the anamnesis and essentially when there is a correlation between a frustrating environmental event and the onset of the alteration.

➤ Exclusion of any underlying medical problems: this involves carrying out the pertinent differential diagnostic tests to rule out possible clinical conditions and reach a diagnosis of exclusion.

➤ Differential diagnosis for flea allergy dermatitis (FAD), food allergies, atopic dermatitis, anal sacculitis, spinal cord injuries, feline lower urinary tract disease (FLUTD), constipation, etc.

➤ Rule out subclinical temporal lobe epilepsy by conducting an electroencephalogram. Antiepileptic drugs can achieve therapeutic success quickly, but anticonvulsive therapy should not be initiated without ensuring the patient has subclinical epilepsy through an electroencephalogram.

TREATMENT

➤ **Behavioural therapy:** while behaviour modification techniques are useful, they are not as helpful as in other behavioural disorders because cats with hyperaesthesia become overexcited and scared making them very hard to handle. Systematic desensitisation and counterconditioning are used to teach the animal to withstand the stimuli that trigger its behaviour and therefore decrease its level of excitation.

➤ **Environmental modification**: it is essential to eliminate the cause of the stress. Environmental enrichment helps transform suboptimal surroundings into an acceptable setting for the animal. Remember that owners form part of the environment, so if the vet notices an owner handling their animal or the situation inappropriately, they should correct this.

➤ **Drug treatment** within the indicated therapeutic range.
  - ➤ Clonazepam*: 0.25–1.10 mg/cat, every 12 h, orally.
  - ➤ Buspirone*: 1–5 mg/cat/day, split over two doses, orally.
  - ➤ Amitriptyline: 5–10 mg/cat, every 24 h, orally.
  - ➤ Clomipramine: 0.5–1.5 mg/cat, every 24 h, orally.
  - ➤ Phenobarbital: 2–3 mg/kg, every 8 h, orally.
  - ➤ Prednisone: 1–2 mg/kg, every 48 h, orally, for 10 days.
  - ➤ Fluoxetine*: 0.5–1.0 mg/kg, every 24 h, orally.
  - ➤ Megestrol acetate: 2.5–10.0 mg/cat, every 24 h, orally, reduce the initial dose progressively.

This list includes some drugs indicated for the treatment of clinical conditions that bear an influence on hyperaesthesia (e.g. corticosteroids, barbiturates, hormonal drugs) or which are used to make differential diagnoses and have been reported as useful in certain cases treated by different authors.

WOOL SUCKING

ANAMNESIS

In this disorder, more specific information can be collected during the anamnesis, particularly regarding the breed, as wool sucking is generally seen in oriental breeds and especially in Siamese and Siamese cross breeds.

➤ Environmental changes related with the appearance of the problem: although environmental factors are not as influential in this disorder as with the previous compulsive behaviours, since the genetic factor assumes a more prominent role in the manifestation of wool sucking (which occurs in kittens), their importance should not be neglected because an impoverished environment can trigger the behaviour in genetically predisposed animals.

➤ Other behavioural problems: do not rule out the possibility of other behavioural disorders; like many other diseases, animal behavioural problems almost always course concomitantly with other morbid

* The author's preferred drugs, but they are not the only viable options available.

conditions, and in the particular case of wool sucking, they can guide vets to the correct diagnosis and treatment.

➤ Observation of the animal and its relationship with its owner: to determine if the owner is reinforcing the cat's behaviour. The main indication is very obvious; each time the animal has access to wool or other fabrics (usually materials with lanolin) to suck on, and although the origin is mainly genetic, the owner may often induce the cat to exhibit the behaviour due to a lack of attention. Therefore, it associates wool sucking with contact with its owner, even if it is in the form of punishment. So, the cat should not be punished, but rather distracted.

DIAGNOSIS

Diagnosis is based on:

➤ Information gathered during the anamnesis and through direct observation.

➤ Differential diagnosis of other food-related behavioural disorders such as pica and polyphagia.

➤ Breed: oriental breeds in general and particularly Siamese cats.

➤ Tendency to suck other fabrics, generally those which contain lanolin.

TREATMENT

➤ **Behavioural therapy**: distraction techniques. It is very important to avoid direct punishment and reinforcing the behaviour, if that is occurring.

➤ **Physically impeding the behaviour**: while a physical barrier (e.g. an Elizabethan collar) is not the appropriate treatment for most compulsive behaviours, it can be useful in the case of wool sucking.

➤ **Drug treatment** within the indicated therapeutic range.

  ➤ Fluoxetine*: 0.5–1.0 mg/kg, every 24 h, orally.
  ➤ Clomipramine: 0.5–1.5 mg/cat, every 24 h, orally.
  ➤ Clonazepam: 0.25–1.10 mg/cat, every 12 h, orally.
  ➤ Buspirone*: 1–5 mg/cat/day, split over two doses, orally.

* The author's preferred drugs, but they are not the only viable options available.

TAIL CHASING WITH OR WITHOUT SELF-MUTILATION

ANAMNESIS

It is important to observe and record the following data during the anamnesis:

➤ The problem behaviour.

➤ The relationship between any significant changes in the animal's environment and the appearance of the anomalous conduct.

➤ Other behavioural disorders: marking, aggression, etc., to obtain a clearer idea of the patient's relationship with its environment (habitat, owner, early life experiences, etc.) and its possible genetic predisposition to abnormal behaviours.

➤ The cat's relationship with its owners: the aim is to learn if the owner is reinforcing the animal's behaviour, whether through punishment or containment by means of stroking, hugs, etc.

DIAGNOSIS

Diagnosis is based on:

➤ Data recorded during the anamnesis and via direct observation of the cat's behaviour and examination of the skin lesions on its tail.

➤ The exclusion of organic conditions, such as tail neuritis, for which an electromyogram of the muscles in the tail region is practically indispensable.

➤ Differential diagnosis between spinal cord injuries, myopathies, neuropathies, etc. Use the necessary complementary methods to this end. The case should be referred to a neurologist to rule out any neurological problems. In addition, if possible, an electroencephalogram should be conducted to rule out the possibility of subclinical epilepsy.

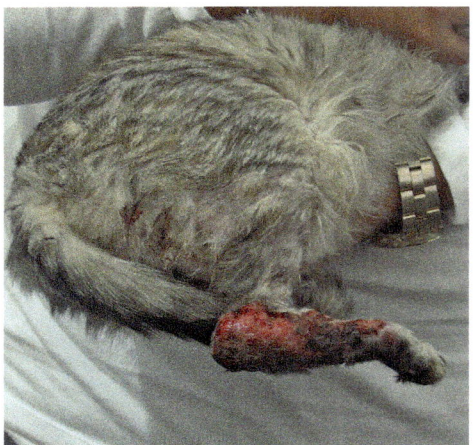

Figure 11. Patient with severe lesions due to licking and self-mutilation.

TREATMENT

- **Behavioural therapy**: remote punishment, behaviour distraction and counterconditioning techniques.
- **Physically impeding the behaviour**: while a physical barrier (e.g. an Elizabethan collar) is not the appropriate treatment for most compulsive behaviours, it can be useful in the case of wool sucking.
- **Environment enrichment**: elimination of stress factors, greater contact with the owner through play, incorporation of another animal (this recommendation must be approved by the owner, as the new animal must be withdrawn from the home if the procedure proves unsuccessful).
- **Drug treatment** within the indicated therapeutic range.
  - Buspirone*: 1–5 mg/cat/day, split over two doses, orally.
  - Fluoxetine*: 0.5–1.0 mg/kg, every 24 h, orally.
  - Clonazepam*: 0.25–1.10 mg/cat, every 12 h, orally.
  - Clomipramine: 0.5–1.5 mg/cat, every 24 h, orally.
  - Phenobarbital: 2–3 mg/kg, every 8 h, orally.
  - Megestrol acetate: 2.5–10.0 mg/cat, every 24 h, orally, reduce the initial dose progressively.

* The author's preferred drugs, but they are not the only viable options available.

PRACTICAL ADVICE

- Rule out clinical problems as the cause of the compulsive disorder. If any do exist, treat the corresponding conditions.
- Observe if the exhibited behaviour is normal for the animal (specific species) and it is just the owner who considers it abnormal.
- Do not give the owner early expectations which could turn out to be false. Stereotypies are behavioural disorders that generally prove hard to resolve, require long-term treatment, and depend heavily on the owner's active participation in the therapeutic strategy, although this is not always feasible for various reasons.
- Are the consequences for the animal severe enough to justify starting treatment? A compulsive behaviour is often the means the cat has discovered to calm its anxiety due to an impoverished environment. For example, a cat that chases imaginary flies when looking out of the window at birds in a tree or an inaccessible cat in the street, will return to its normal life after chasing the nonexistent flies and releasing its anxiety. Assess whether it is really necessary to try and resolve this compulsive behaviour.

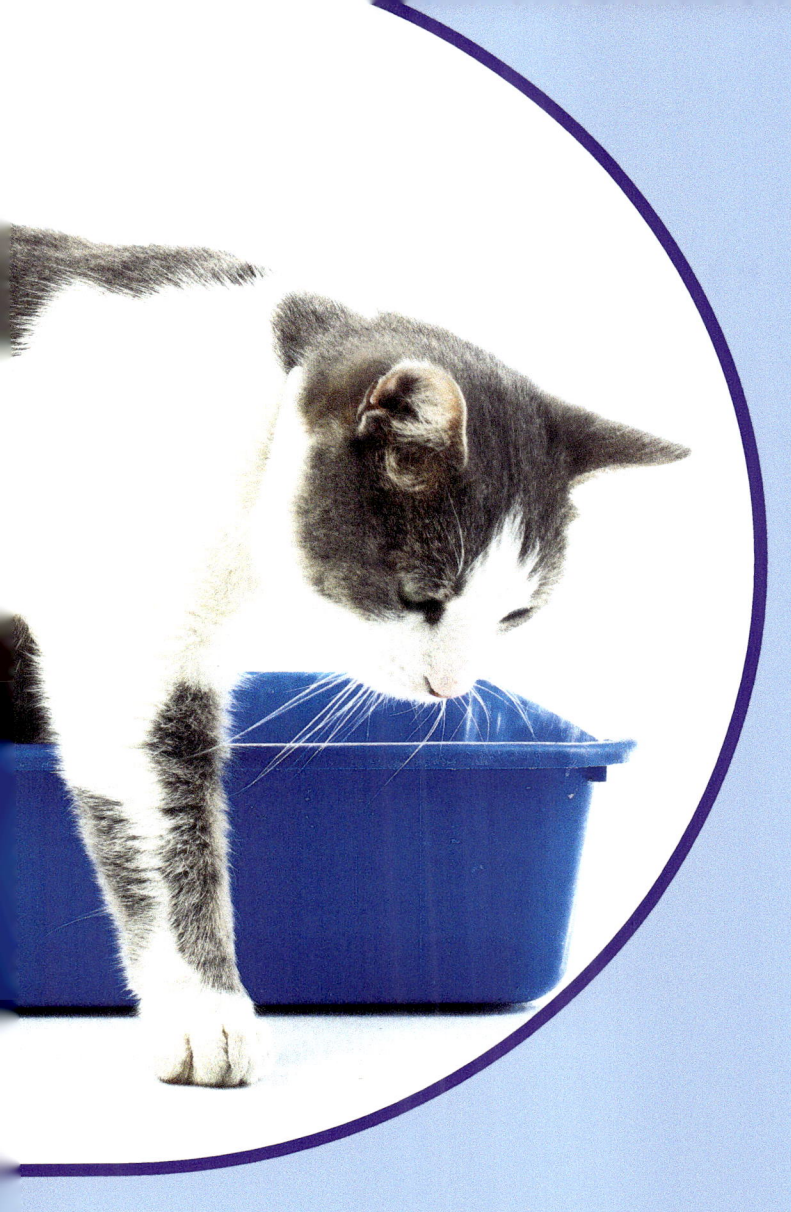

DISORDERS ASSOCIATED WITH ELIMINATION BEHAVIOUR

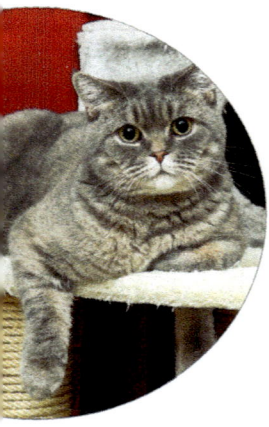

INTRODUCTION

Traditionally, dogs have always been the most popular type of pet in many countries around the world, but in recent years, the popularity of cats has grown enormously. While there are several reasons for their increasing prevalence, the domestic cat's unique elimination behaviour is definitely one of the strongest motives as to why cats are gaining in popularity as household pets, especially among those living in cities.

While cats' orderly elimination behaviour is one of their biggest advantages as a pet, urination or defaecation outside the litter tray constitutes a major problem for owners. Consequently, we can expect consultations for elimination behaviour disorders to be among some of the most frequent complaints associated with behavioural problems in cats. In fact, abnormal elimination conducts are the impetus for 40–70 % of all visits by owners of cats with a behavioural disorder.

Some of the most common elimination behaviour disorders exhibited by domestic cats are those related to inappropriate urination and/or defaecation and urine marking.

In practice, marking is not as typical as inappropriate urination or defaecation, but owners find it a lot harder to accept and more annoying. This is because, as a behaviour normally associated with entire animals, particularly males, the smell of the urine eliminated when marking has a much stronger negative impact on the owner's quality of life than a cat's incorrect use of their litter tray.

> In summary, elimination behaviour disorders exhibited by house cats comprise inappropriate urination or defaecation and marking, mainly urine marking.

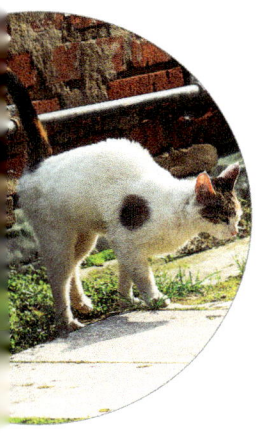

URINE MARKING

Marking behaviour, with or without spraying, is commonly displayed by cats with outdoor access to delimit their territory.

Cats primarily mark vertical surfaces by spraying on them (they assume a standing position with an erect tail). However, they can mark surfaces without spraying or through the use of faeces. In such cases, it is important to differentiate between marking and inappropriate elimination.

In the home, this marking behaviour is typically performed on vertical objects, both indoors (walls, furniture, etc.) and outdoors (trees, wheels, etc.). Cats smell the site where they are about to spray at a height of roughly 30 cm from the ground, then they turn and from a standing position emit a jet of urine, normally just a small volume, onto the surface while holding their tails upright. Although the urine might not be apparent on the vertical surface, the cat may still be eliminating its pungent spray. Some cats will spray on horizontal objects such as beds. In this instance, the urine marked area will not be circular, as occurs with elimination without spraying, but rather it will be elongated.

It is a perfectly normal behaviour for feral street cats, necessary to mark their territory. Marking is more commonplace when intact adult females are present and is further accentuated whenever there is social disorder in the community, in other words, when there are several males competing for the same social range.

> Marking is a serious problem for owners of cats with no outdoor access and is one of the principal behavioural disorders that vets are asked to help resolve in cats.

It is easily distinguished from inappropriate urination because when marking cats urinate perpendicularly to the object being sprayed, at a height of 30 cm from the ground, while standing still and with an erect tail, and they do not subsequently scratch the surface (Fig. 1). Inappropriate urination, however, involves voiding in an unacceptable location while assuming a crouched position with a lowered tail and the cat will urinate perpendicular to the floor (Fig. 2).

Another significant difference is the amount of urine the animal voids, which is approximately 1 mL when marking and around 20 mL in the case of inappropriate elimination.

Besides discerning between the two behaviours, it is also important to learn why the conduct has arisen. Cats generally tend to start marking because of a temporary environmental situation, yet they may persist with the habit even when the cause is no longer present.

Some of the most common aetiological factors, apart from hormones, are the arrival of a new member of the household, moving to a new house, disproportionate punishment by the owner, the presence of a new cat in the neighbourhood that is marking just outside the cat's home, and so on.

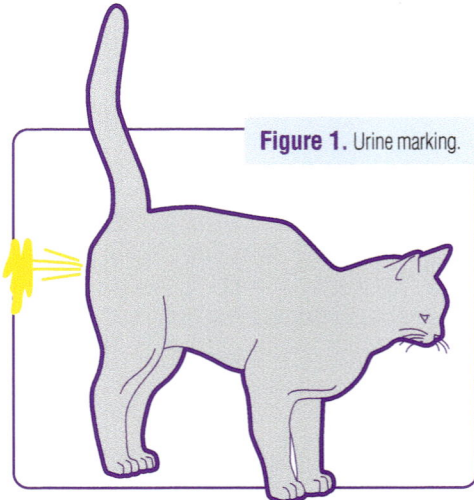

Figure 1. Urine marking.

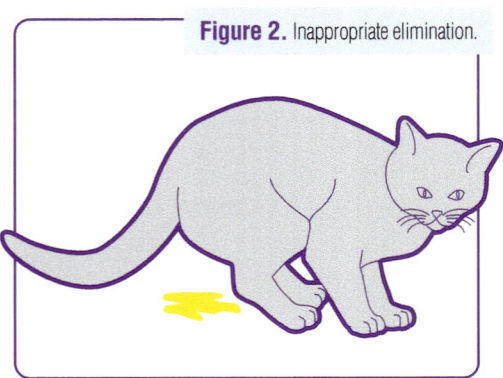

Figure 2. Inappropriate elimination.

➤ Marking without spraying

Marking behaviour, with or without spraying, is often used by cats with outdoor access to delimit their territory. Cats can still mark surfaces without spraying by means of their urine or faeces. Feral cats usually employ various methods to mark their territorial boundary.

If strange or unknown cats are passing close to the front door and the cat living inside the house urinates or defaecates next to this door, in addition to in its litter tray, then this is almost definitely a marking behaviour. The same may occur in a multicat household; the owner may notice that one or more cats start to eliminate their waste in inappropriate locations following a change in social relationships or the arrival of a new cat.

➤ Marking with spraying

Urine spraying is primarily exhibited by entire males after they have reached sexual maturity. However, since the behavioural differences between males and females are quantitative and not qualitative, both castrated and intact females as well as castrated males also manifest marking behaviours, although less frequently. Urine spraying forms part of normal cat behaviour and is regulated and activated by androgens, although oestrogens also contribute to the emergence of this behaviour. Different studies indicate that urine spraying is not just influenced by hormonal components, but also by social and territorial factors where it serves for communication purposes. While it is true that cats mainly spray urine during the breeding season to attract members of the opposite sex, they also spray outside this period for the reasons given previously. Marking with spraying serves other functions as well: to delimit and familiarise itself with its territory, to organise and defend its territory, and to act as a means of communication with other cats (Figs. 3 and 4).

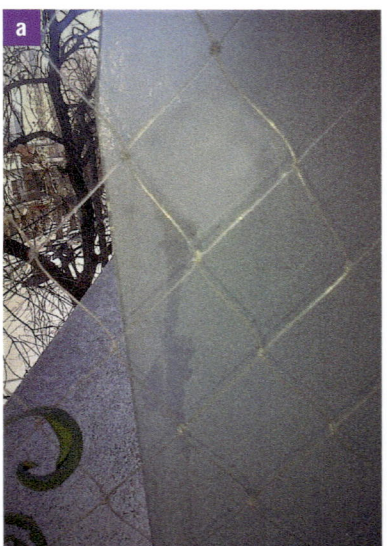 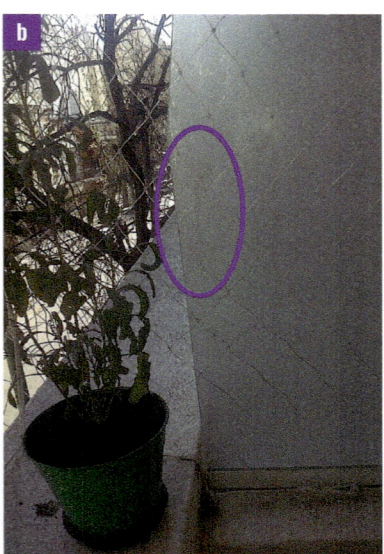

Figure 3. Urine marking carried out on a wall (a). Note the height of the marking (b).

DIAGNOSIS

The medical causes associated with the onset of this behaviour include both functional and organic factors.

➤ Functional: deterritorialisation anxiety and stress due to environmental frustration.

➤ Organic: cognitive dysfunction syndrome, which is very common among very elderly cats.

Urine marking is diagnosed by inspecting the cat's living environment and based on information collected from the owner during the anamnesis. The diagnosis is relatively straightforward, but it is much harder to give a prognosis about how long it will take to resolve the problem and the inauguration of the corresponding medical treatment. The main parameter indicative of a diagnosis of urine marking is the amount of urine voided; cats eliminate approximately 1 mL of urine when marking, which is a lot less than the volume expelled during normal urination of about 20 mL.

However, it is considerably harder to make a correct diagnosis when several cats live in the same household and the owner is unable to identify which cat is spraying inside the home. In this case, the anamnesis is vital to the diagnosis (e.g. which was the last cat to join the household, what are the different attitudes exhibited by the cats, what is the hormonal status of each cat, etc.). In more complicated cases, the administration of dyes (fluorescein) is indicated to stain the urine and identify which cat is marking around the home. However, this diagnostic technique is only necessary in a very limited number of cases.

DIFFERENTIAL DIAGNOSIS

It is crucial to differentiate between urine marking and cats that have developed an aversion or preference for a given location or surface. Therefore, one of the most important aspects to consider is the location where the cat is voiding. If the urination sites are closely linked to an external factor (doors and windows), it is most likely due to a marking behaviour. If, on the other hand, the location of choice is isolated or in a sheltered area and the cat voids a relatively large volume of urine, then it is probably a case of inappropriate elimination. Another point to bear in mind is the social element. For example, if the elimination disorder emerges due to a change in the individual's social group, it is almost certainly an instance of a urine marking behaviour. Figure 4 can aid in the diagnostic process. It features the possible causes of urine marking or situations that may result in inappropriate elimination behaviour based upon the cat's posture when urinating.

> Urine marking behaviour in cats depends on the subject's plasma concentrations of sex hormones, the level of stress or anxiety to which they are exposed, and any external influences from their surrounding environment.

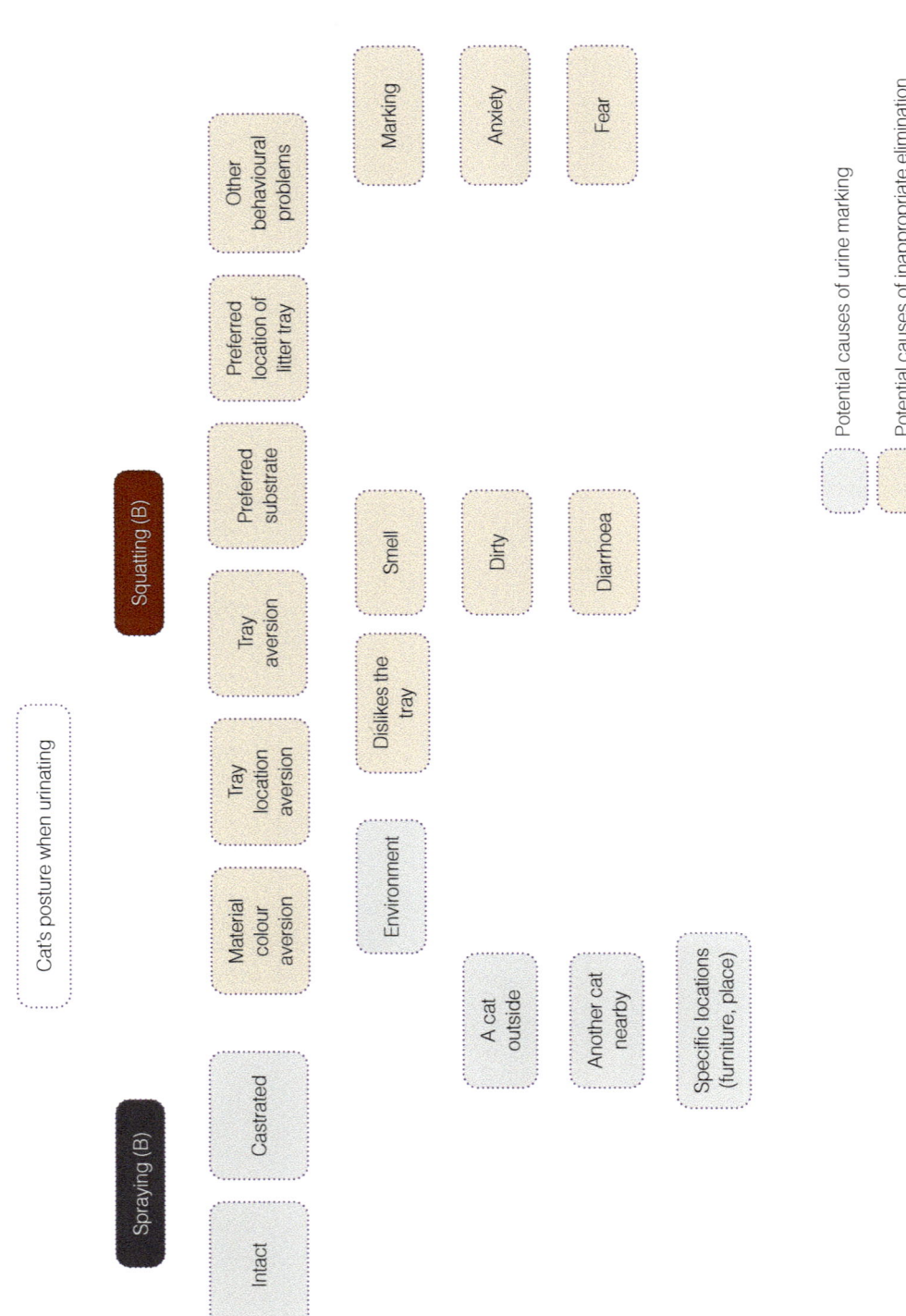

Figure 4. Possible causes of urine marking or inappropriate elimination behaviours.

PROGNOSIS

The prognosis largely depends on the correct diagnosis of the case. Therapeutic success is generally achieved quickly and at a high rate, provided that the cause of the problem behaviour has been diagnosed, so cases only require a short follow-up period. If psychoactive drugs are necessary, veterinary surgeons must keep in touch with the patient's owner throughout the follow-up.

PREVENTION

Prevention involves managing the patient correctly and awareness of the specific behavioural patterns of household cats. The two main points to consider are to avoid overcrowding and make sure the introduction of new members to a well-balanced social group is carried out correctly. For example, new cats can be housed in a cage for one or two days to let them get used to their new home, while the other animals can familiarise themselves with their new housemate.

TREATMENT

The treatment of choice will depend on the underlying cause of the cat's behavioural problem. If there is a confirmed medical cause, its treatment must be taken as the starting point for behaviour therapy.

If the cat has not been castrated, and the owner agrees, the first treatment to recommend should be castration, which would also eradicate the pungent odour of urine left by entire male cats. Castration is a surgical procedure with an efficacy of 80 %.

The behavioural management of the case is very important. Owners must reduce any stress- or anxiety-inducing factors and clean urine marked areas with a 25 % solution of white vinegar. Additionally, environmental enrichment, granting the cat more time outside, and strategic space management (areas for resting and feeding) are essential considerations.

It is important to advise the owner against physical punishment, as this can produce fear or anxiety, which will make the cat exhibit the undesired behaviour more frequently, thereby perpetuating the problem as the cat–owner relationship will start to deteriorate. Punishment is only indicated if the owner catches their pet in the act of marking a surface with urine, which is actually quite rare because they rapidly learn not to mark when their owners are nearby. A water pistol or compressed air spray make ideal punishments to help correct marking behaviour, but remember they must only be used exactly in the moment the cat is performing the inappropriate action.

If the cat always sprays on the same object, placing a material on the floor around the object which the cat does not like to walk on, such as aluminium foil, can be very helpful. There are also special devices available equipped with a light sensor and which emit an unpleasant smell (e.g. limonene) for any cats that come to close.

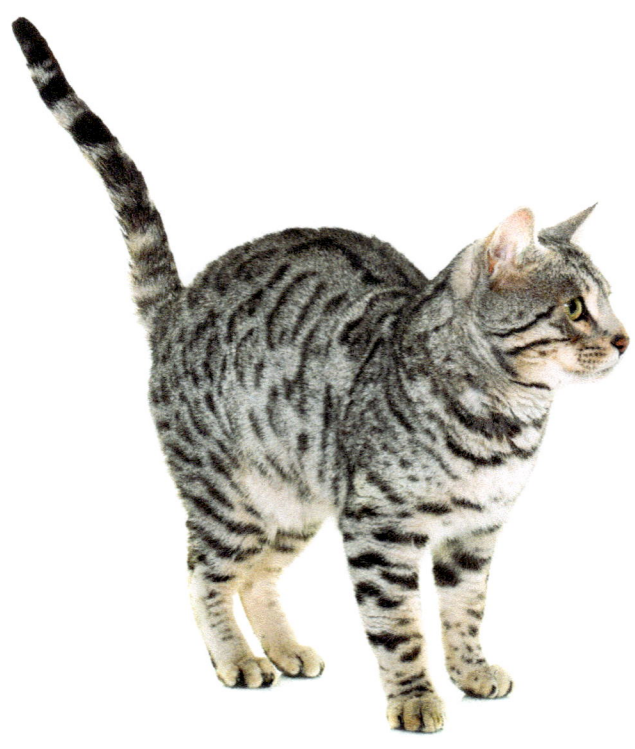

Regarding drug treatment, as with other behavioural disorders in cats, vets are advised to prescribe nonbenzodiazepine anxiolytic agents such as buspirone and selective serotonin reuptake inhibitors (SSRI) such as fluoxetine.

Some studies have shown that vasopressin (the neurotransmitter involved in regulating urine marking) antagonists reduce the frequency of this behaviour. In stressful situations, neurons in the hypothalamus release vasopressin. Serotonin inhibits neuronal vasopressin production, so drugs that affect serotonin regulation (SSRI) are useful in the treatment of urine marking in cats.

Another option is the use of commercially available cat pheromones which contain a synthetic analogue of the F3 fraction of natural feline pheromones.

If these treatments do not work, another weapon in the therapeutic arsenal is the administration of progestogens:
➤ Medroxyprogesterone acetate: 100 mg in total in males, 50 mg in total in castrated females, administered intramuscularly.
➤ Megestrol acetate: 2.5–10.0 mg/day given orally, followed by gradual reduction at 1 or 2 week intervals down to a dose of 5.0 mg once a week for a maximum of 2 or 3 months.

Owners should respect their cat's circadian rhythm, so this type of medication should be administered in the evening, sometime after 6 p.m. Vets must assess the use of this hormone therapy, particularly in females, and weigh up its potential advantages against possible side effects. Veterinary professionals should advise owners to confine their cat in a suitable location while receiving medical treatment, make them aware of the possible side effects of progestogen hormone therapy, and perform blood tests before and after its administration.

According to statistics, hormone therapy has a 30 % success rate in animals that do not respond satisfactorily to surgical treatment, which underlines the importance of identifying the origin of the behaviour and not simply assuming that it is an exclusively hormone-related problem.

Anxiolytics are of great help, mainly in cases where the patient has been diagnosed as suffering from anxiety. Buspirone hydrochloride is the treatment of choice in such cases thanks to its efficacy and the low probability of side effects.

➤ Buspirone: 1–5 mg/cat/day, split over two doses, orally.

➤ Fluoxetine: 0.5–1.0 mg/kg, every 24 h.

➤ Megestrol acetate: 2.5–10.0 mg/cat/day, reduce the initial dose progressively.

Finally, olfactory tractotomy is a neurosurgical treatment that has demonstrated success rates of 50 % in males and almost 100 % in females. The procedure eradicates the patient's sense of smell and is only indicated for cats that are refractory to aforementioned therapeutic measures and as a last resort as opposed to euthanasia (something which owners often request because they can no longer tolerate their pet's behavioural disorder).

MARKING AND AGGRESSION

Urine marking behaviour has very important social and hormonal components. In addition, among its distinct functions, communication is particularly relevant. So, it is important to bear in mind that marking can manifest in tandem with aggressive behaviour. In such cases, vets must assess the risk to the physical integrity of any individuals affected by said behaviour.

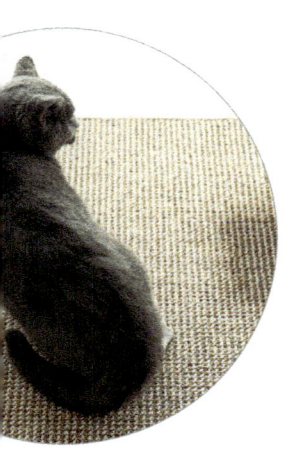

INAPPROPRIATE ELIMINATION

Inappropriate elimination is characterised by cats urinating (usually in large quantities) or defaecating outside their litter trays, either directly on the floor or other horizontal surfaces, and after turning around in circles and taking up a crouching position, before finally trying to cover their waste.

Several factors contribute to this behaviour. Cats are very sensitive to environmental changes such as the appearance of other animals or people in the house, a decline in the cat–owner relationship, relocation to a new home, among others, and such environmental factors can trigger inappropriate elimination.

Cats are extremely clean and scrupulous, qualities that they have developed through natural selection to help them adapt to their habitat and control diseases, particularly those borne by parasites. They shun away from contaminated areas, so if owners do not keep the litter tray clean their pet cats will start to use other locations. Even when provided with a clean litter tray, the cat may sometimes still eliminate its waste elsewhere, although it will eventually correct this conduct.

Older cats that have always used their tray but suddenly start voiding outside it almost certainly have an underlying pathophysiological problem. For example, an episode of painful diarrhoea, cystitis, or kidney stones can produce a negative association between the painful event and the litter tray or substrate. This tray–pain association may persist even after resolving the medical problem, so the cat will continue to exhibit the behavioural disorder.

Borchelt published a communication in which he reported treating a disproportionate number of Persian cats with inappropriate elimination outside the litter tray, indicating a clear genetic influence over this behavioural problem.

DIAGNOSIS

It is important to focus on the information gathered from the anamnesis, as cats can develop an aversion to litter trays, the substrate, or the tray's location.

Aversion can emerge suddenly, following a traumatic experience, or gradually, due to regular exposure to unpleasant situations.

BEHAVIOURAL DISORDERS IN CATS

When a cat starts to eliminate its waste in inappropriate places, it can prove very hard to establish whether it has developed an aversion or, conversely, a preference for a new location or substrate. There are even occasions where the problem is initially caused by one stimulus but perpetuated by a totally different one. As a case in point, a cat may change its elimination site due to an aversion to the substrate and later develop a preference for another location or substrate (the earth in a plant pot, for example); so even though the original cause is addressed, the cat may continue to exhibit the behaviour because the stimulus for which it has developed a preference is still present. There are various types of aversion which can arise from different situations and stimuli.

➤ Aversion to tray location: some of the most common causes include placing the tray in busy areas, locations associated with the presence of an individual the cat does not like (dogs, another cat, certain humans, etc.), in the vicinity of household appliances with a timer (e.g. washing machines, dishwashers), or in the same place as where the cat feeds or plays.

➤ Aversion to the tray: this aversion is often connected to the size of the tray (too small) or the height of its edges, whether too high or too low.

➤ Aversion to the substrate: the animal dislikes the material used in the litter tray. Cats are very sensitive to changes, especially abrupt changes, and very meticulous when it comes to their elimination habits, so it is essential to keep the tray clean and replace the substrate frequently. When multiple cats share the same house, it is imperative that they have an adequate number of litter trays. Cats can develop an aversion due to a causal association (e.g. a substrate with a very hard texture in the case of cats with injured paws or which have suffered dysuria or diarrhoea and associate the pain caused by these illnesses with the litter tray material) or noncausal association with a pain-inducing stimulus (such as organic diseases that course with pain).

> There are many other causes related to the substrate that can result in an aversion: uncleanliness, moisture, strong odours noted by the cat, the smell of an unwell animal that has used the tray, a substrate with a hard texture or excessively large granules, etc.

House cats are known to develop preferences for a given substrate for urination, defaecation, or both. This means some cats may start urinating outside their tray but still continue defaecating in it. The development of a preference may or may not be accompanied by the generation of an aversion. When this happens, the preference for the new substrate manifests after the appearance of the aversion.

Regardless of how the preference becomes apparent, cats tend to choose fine substrates with a soft texture. Any owner whose cat has, at some time, had access to sand will have almost certainly noticed this preference. So, given the choice, cats usually eliminate their waste on sand, particularly urine. This predilection for a soft material seems to be innate, as it is similar to the substrates used by the domestic cat's evolutionary ancestor – the African wildcat (*Felis libyca*).

Various studies into cats with an inappropriate elimination disorder have shown that long-haired breeds are more likely to develop a substrate preference than short-haired cats.

Cats typically develop a preference for a new location because a social problem has emerged. They tend to prefer quiet locations to void their waste, so they will look for a new elimination site if there is too much activity around their current location. Individuals that live in multicat households will often try to find a new location if they feel overwhelmed by their feline housemates. In these cases, it can be difficult to distinguish between inappropriate elimination and urine marking. For the former, the new site will generally be an isolated location where the cat feels protected (Fig. 5).

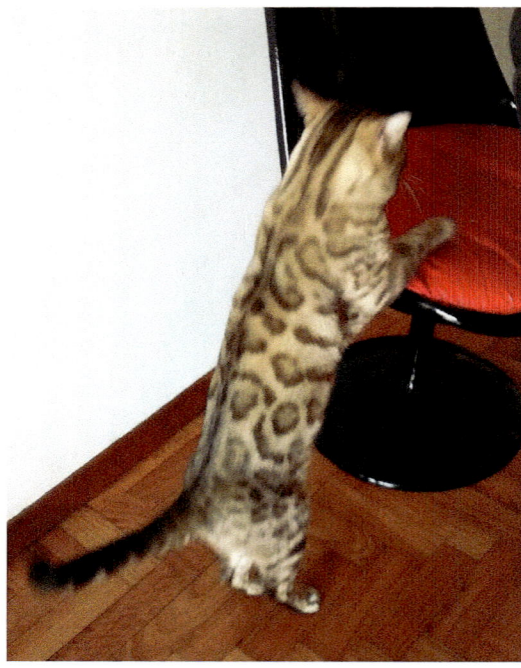

Figure 5. This cat is just about to jump onto and then urinate on its owner's chair, a behaviour it did regularly, and which compelled the owner to seek their vet's advice.

The first step in the diagnosis is to rule out the possibility of a somatic condition. A thorough clinical examination is therefore necessary and complementary studies (blood chemistry and urinalysis) should be conducted based on professional judgement.

Important signs in the diagnosis of inappropriate elimination behaviour are:
1. The elimination posture the cat adopts when urinating in an unacceptable location. In cases of inappropriate elimination, the cat will void while crouching, with its tail down and parallel to the floor, and later try to cover the urine or faeces by scratching the ground.
2. Urine volume. Cats void a much larger volume of urine in comparison with cases of urine marking. In inappropriate elimination, cats will expel approximately 20 mL of urine.

When several cats are living together, the owner will have to determine which individual is eliminating inappropriately. As a first recourse, vets should carry out a thorough anamnesis and base their conclusions on the data provided by the patient's owner. If this is not possible, the cat can be given fluorescein which will be eliminated in their urine after 2 hours and lasts for up to 24 hours on the surfaces where it urinates. Veterinary professionals should administer a 10 % fluorescein solution, either 0.3 mL subcutaneously or 0.5 mL orally, to the most suspicious cat. If it turns out that the first cat is not responsible for the behaviour, the same solution should be given to another cat after 48 hours, and so on, until the culprit is identified. Owners may sometimes need to use a Wood's lamp to detect the presence of the fluorescein.

A differential diagnosis is normally made between inappropriate elimination and urine marking (Fig. 4).

MEDICAL CAUSES

Various medical problems, both organic and functional, can cause or contribute to inappropriate elimination behaviours. So, besides a thorough clinical examination, vets must also request complementary studies such as urine and stool analyses.

➤ Inappropriate urination: this behaviour can be a clinical sign of several different medical conditions including cystitis, ectopic ureter, diabetes *mellitus*, feline lower urinary tract disease, cognitive dysfunction syndrome, musculoskeletal disorders, anxiety, phobias, and depression.

➤ Inappropriate defaecation: this undesired conduct may be secondary to constipation, diarrhoea, parasites, cognitive dysfunction syndrome, musculoskeletal disorders, anxiety, phobias, etcetera.

PROGNOSIS

Cases of inappropriate elimination should receive monthly follow-ups, particularly if the treatment includes psychoactive drugs.

Prevention consists of placing the litter tray in a suitable location, ensuring there are enough trays according to the number of cats, and selecting the correct substrate based on the cat's preference.

It is fundamental that attempts are made to correct this behavioural disorder as soon as possible, since it will take longer to rectify the problem the longer it is allowed to occur.

In most cases, the problem can be resolved quickly following a correct differential diagnosis, so follow-up often only requires one or two subsequent visits.

> The prognosis is generally favourable in terms of the chances of success and the eradication of the patient's unwanted behaviour.

TREATMENT

Treatment of choice depends on the cause of the problem. Owners should be given advice on the proper usage of litter trays (location, substrate, and cleaning), how to identify the origin of the problem (poor cat–owner relationship, stress due to environmental changes, clinical problems, unsuitable choice of litter tray location or material, etc.), and how to retrain their pet without using any physical punishment but instead discouraging the behaviour from afar in the exact moment the cat is voiding inappropriately, while also rewarding any appropriate behaviour.

If there is an underlying medical cause, any therapeutic plan must first aim to treat this organic problem before tackling the behavioural problem.

MEASURES THAT CAN HELP RESOLVE INAPPROPRIATE ELIMINATION BEHAVIOUR

➤ Intervene in the olfactory component: clean the areas marked with the animal's urine using a 25 % solution of white vinegar.
➤ Change the texture or type of litter tray substrate.
➤ Try aversive conditioning in the area where the patient is exhibiting the inappropriate elimination.
➤ Strategic space management: impede the cat's access to the areas where it performs inappropriate elimination.
➤ Strategic management of rest and feeding areas: cats always keep these areas clean, so they will not use litter trays if placed nearby.
➤ Place the tray in a suitable location (isolated, quiet, private, etc.).
➤ Provide enough trays in the case of multicat households.
➤ Retrain cats that have developed this behavioural problem.
➤ Keep the tray clean and replace the substrate based on the patient's individual characteristics (some cats are fussier than others when it comes to the cleanliness of their tray).

With regard to drug therapy, recommendations are for nonbenzodiazepine anxiolytics and selective serotonin reuptake inhibitors, although other drugs have been indicated in the literature and recommended by other authors:

➤ Buspirone: 1–5 mg/cat/day, split over two doses, orally.
➤ Fluoxetine: 0.5–1.0 mg/kg, every 24 h, orally.
➤ Amitriptyline: 0.5–1.0 mg/kg/day, in one or two oral doses.
➤ Clomipramine: 0.5–1.0 mg/kg/day, in one or two oral doses.

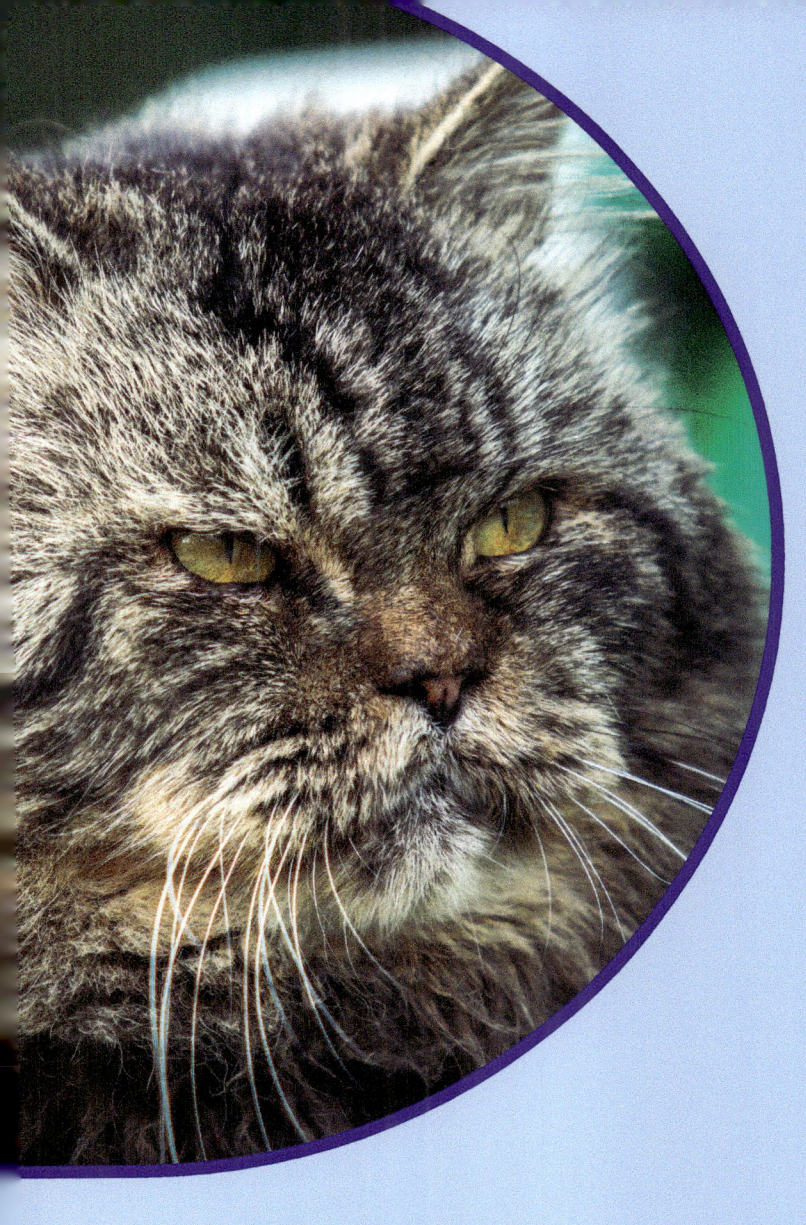

LESS COMMON DISORDERS
SEEN IN EVERYDAY PRACTICE

INTRODUCTION

Although the behavioural disorders explained in this chapter do not arise very often in everyday practice, they are still worthy of at least some discussion, as knowledge of their existence will allow veterinary professionals to make better differential diagnoses and therefore improve their overall performance in behavioural consultations.

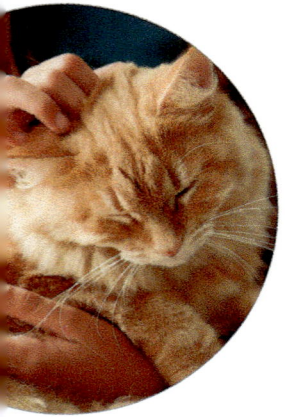

SYNDROMES ASSOCIATED WITH COGNITIVE DECLINE

Fortunately, veterinary medicine started to pay attention to geriatric care quite some time ago. Animal behaviour most certainly cannot and should not be excluded from this situation. Within this specialised area, cognitive dysfunction syndrome (CDS) is one of the main behavioural disorders observed in geriatric animals.

DIAGNOSIS

It is vital that we recognise elderly cats aged 12–15 years are no longer adults, but rather should be considered geriatric patients, in order to make a correct diagnosis. In behavioural terms, domestic animals go through significant organic changes in old age and, unlike other veterinary specialities, in ethology there is an additional factor to consider in elderly animals – the difficulty owners experience in changing their own behaviours and routines with respect to how they treat their pets in this distinct stage of their lives. As animals enter into old age, they suffer neurochemical and vascular changes in the brain which can produce cognitive deficits that consequently cause the animal to exhibit abnormal or different behaviours compared to when they were adults.

The natural degeneration of the animal's different organ systems also has a very strong impact:

➤ Osteoarticular disorders (arthritis, spondylosis, etc.): that are painful for the animal and increase the likelihood of an aggressive response when disturbed.

➤ Urogenital problems (cystitis, prostatomegaly, kidney failure, etc.): can make the animal neglect the elimination habits it has learned over the years.

➤ Liver diseases: these can induce a state of autointoxication that in turn contributes to neurological disorders associated with behavioural alterations.

There are a lot more examples, since any organic dysfunction, in one way or another, may affect the animal's behaviour.

> It has been shown that animal dementia is accompanied by the same changes in brain chemistry that occur in humans suffering from Alzheimer's disease and senile dementia.

Such alterations can be treated, but not cured, with drugs similar to those used in human medicine (nicergoline, L-deprenyl, propentofylline, etc.).

Focusing on cats, the main reasons for consultation are:

➤ Urine marking or inappropriate elimination (spraying furniture with urine or urinating somewhere other than the litter tray).

➤ Aggression directed towards other animals or people.

➤ Alterations associated with heightened states of anxiety (vocalisation, phobias, ingestion of foreign objects such as clothes, wool, pieces of wood, etc.).

BEHAVIOURAL DISORDERS IN CATS

Another point worth considering is that elderly animals experience a decline in their overall sensory capacity, although they mainly suffer a progressive loss of sight and hearing. This loss contributes to a greater level of anxiety, since the animal is stressed as a result of the insecurity it feels in day-to-day situations. For example, a diminished sense of space and time can mean cats start to urinate anywhere. If owners scold or punish their cats when they find the urine or faeces, it will instil more stress and anxiety and the cat will respond by displaying other undesired conducts that in turn cause further deterioration of the cat–owner relationship.

Veterinary surgeons must take all these factors into account to arrive at a professional and accurate diagnosis of each case.

PROGNOSIS

These cases should always be given a guarded prognosis, since the primary cause of the behavioural disorder is treatable but not curable, so vets must explain the situation to the patient's owner with particular caution.

TREATMENT

> The role and participation of owners is crucial in both the origin and treatment of these syndromes.

The main contributing factor to behavioural alterations in elderly animals, regardless of the organic changes typically observed in old age, is that owners do not always realise or accept that their pet is growing or has grown old, a point that is reflected in their resistance to become the primary actors in the animal's treatment. Therefore, broadly speaking, treatment consists of drug therapy, correct management by the owner, and behavioural therapy (Fig. 1).

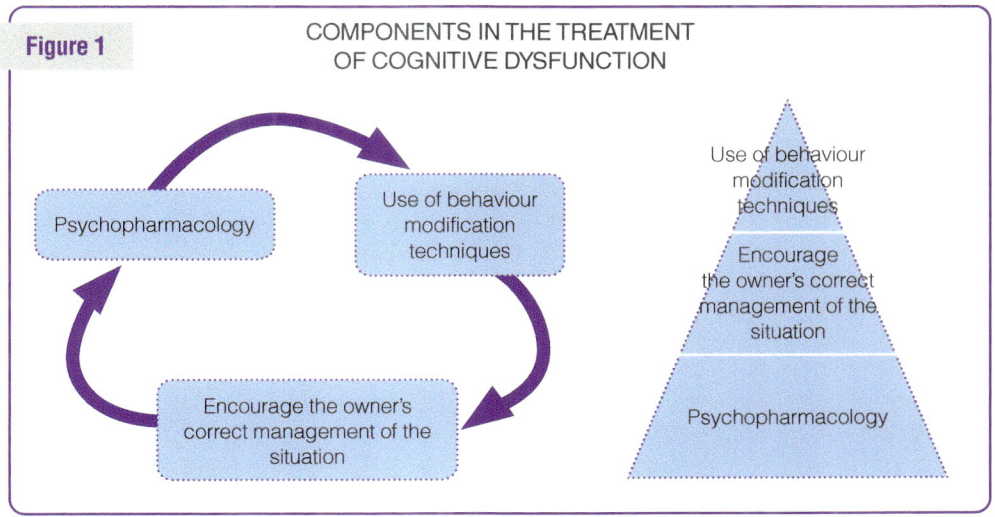

Figure 1

COMPONENTS IN THE TREATMENT
OF COGNITIVE DYSFUNCTION

Psychopharmacology

Use of behaviour
modification
techniques

Encourage the owner's
correct management of the
situation

Use of behaviour
modification
techniques

Encourage
the owner's correct
management of the
situation

Psychopharmacology

➤ **Drug treatment**

   ➤ Propentofylline: a new therapeutic agent for the treatment of dementia that crosses the blood–brain barrier easily and acts by blocking
adenosine reuptake and inhibiting the enzyme phosphodiesterase.
It has a dual mechanism of action: it inhibits free radical production
and reduces microglial cell activation. This means it interacts with the
inflammatory processes that contribute to dementia and, thanks to its
mechanism of action, potentially modifies the disease rather than offer-
ing a purely symptomatic treatment. A rough dose range is 3–5 mg/kg,
twice a day, orally.

   ➤ Citicoline: improves brain function and metabolism, thus promoting
glucose reuptake and inhibiting lactic acid buildup in the brain and
fatty acid radicalisation in cerebral ischaemia. It should be administered orally as a total dose of 50 mg split over two daily doses.

   ➤ Selegiline: inhibits monoamine oxidase-B (MAO-B) and therefore
reduces dopamine metabolism. Selegiline promotes superoxide dis-
mutase activity, thus contributes to the capture of free radicals, which
accelerate cell ageing. This helps limit the amount of neuronal death
and consequent release of even more free radicals. It also improves lipid
bilayer fluidity during synaptic transmission. It can be administered at
a dosage of 5 mg/day split over two oral doses.

➤ Nicergoline: belongs to the ergoline group of compounds (synthetic analogues of natural ergot alkaloids with sympatholytic properties). It is an alpha-adrenergic receptor blocking agent with cerebral vasodilator activity. It has a vasodilatory action and stimulates metabolism. Nicergoline acts on dopamine D2 receptors in the mesolimbic system and in the striatum, which increases cerebral dopamine production and reduces prolactin production. It also promotes cerebral norepinephrine production with a greater affinity for alpha-1 adrenergic receptors. Furthermore, it improves ion flow speeds, increases cerebral blood flow, especially in hypoperfused areas, and inhibits platelet agglutination, which improves blood viscosity. Nicergoline is administered orally at a rate of 0.25–0.50 mg/kg/day.

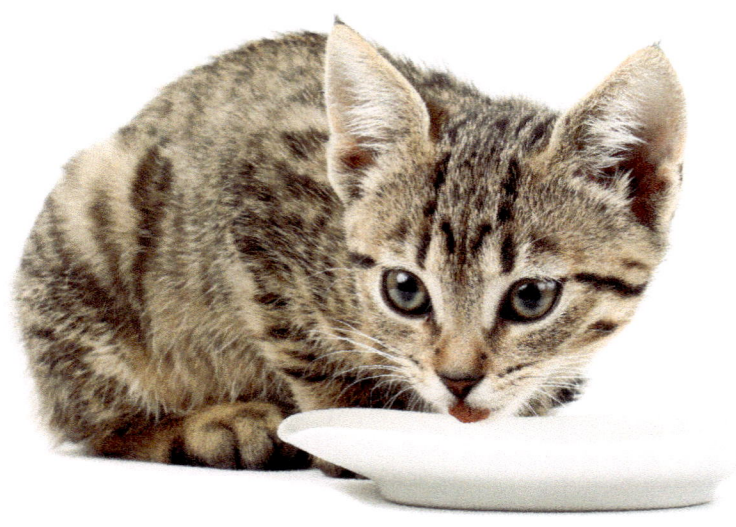

➤ **Behavioural therapy**
  - ➤ Environmental enrichment of the cat's surroundings.
  - ➤ Encourage the cat to be as active as possible.
  - ➤ Leave a light on at night to compensate for the elderly cat's possible vision loss.
  - ➤ Owners must adapt how they treat their cat in line with its age.

WHAT DO OWNERS NEED TO UNDERSTAND ABOUT THEIR ELDERLY CAT?

Vets should ensure that owners of elderly pets remember that geriatric animals rest nearly all day long and are only physically active for brief periods.

In short, we must help them appreciate and accept that their pet is no longer, or will soon cease to be, the animal it once was and is entering into a stage in which the owner should repay the companionship they have received throughout the cat's life with understanding, patience, and care to make sure it enjoys the best possible quality of life until its final days.

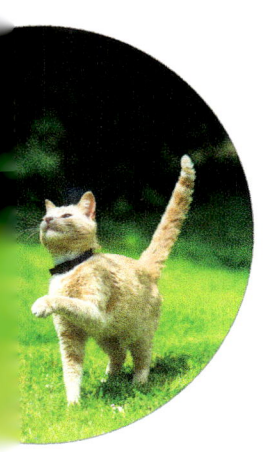

VAGRANCY

It is hard to categorise vagrancy as a behavioural disorder in cats, since it is a completely normal conduct even for house cats; nevertheless, despite this, many owners still want to modify the behaviour.

DIAGNOSIS

The diagnosis is quite straightforward and based on information reported by owners. Most cats that exhibit vagrancy are outdoor cats, that is, they can access and explore their neighbourhood. Cats generally start to become restless at around 6 or 7 p.m. and often energetically and continuously vocalise until they are let out of the house. Such cats normally pass the whole night outside and return in the early morning, which often causes anxiety for the owner. This behaviour is much more common and evident among males compared to females and even more so in the case of intact and castrated males. Cats that roam around tend to fight with other cats and may often display the physical signs of these fights (e.g. thicker skin on their cheeks). Vagrant house cats are usually quite thin, and their coat is poorly cared for (Fig. 2).

> Vagrancy entails the risk of contracting diseases, many of which can prove fatal for cats.

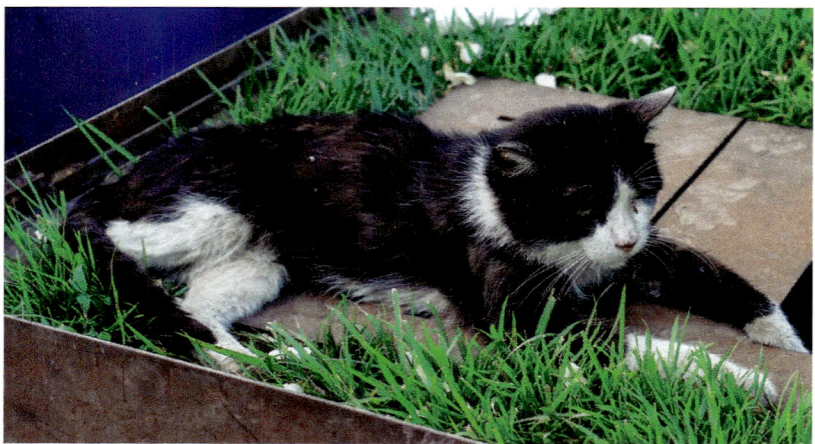

Figure 2. Cats prone to vagrancy are often thin and have an unkempt coat.

PROGNOSIS

The prognosis is generally good because patients will, sooner or later, get used to an indoor lifestyle.

TREATMENT

The treatment of choice is surgical castration for entire male cats. If the patient is a previously castrated male or refractory to the first-choice treatment, since it persists with its vagrant behaviour after castration, one option is the oral administration of progestogens and anxiolytic agents to reduce their anxiety. Anxiolytics are also administered when owners agree to deny their cat outdoor access, as this prohibition will initially exacerbate the cat's state of anxiety. In such cases, buspirone and fluoxetine are recommended to treat this anxiety.

➤ Buspirone: 1–5 mg/cat/day, split over two doses, orally.
➤ Fluoxetine: 0.5–1.0 mg/kg, every 24 h, orally.
➤ Megestrol acetate: 2.5–10.0 mg/cat/day, given orally and reduce the initial dose progressively.

> When dealing with female patients, whether intact or castrated, progestogen administration is totally contraindicated as a therapeutic measure because of its potential side effects.

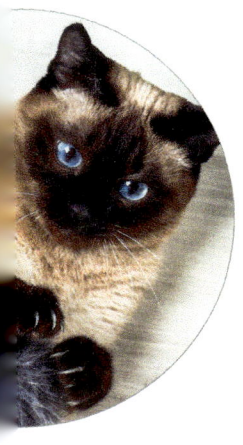

PICA

Pica is defined as eating materials or objects that do not form part of the normal diet for the members of a given species.

In the case cats, they often suck on wool or other textiles. This behaviour is predominantly observed in Siamese cats and their crossbreeds, so some studies have indicated that this group of cats may be affected by a genetic component.

The origin of this disorder seems to be linked to cholecystokinin (CCK) metabolism in the central nervous system (CCK is involved in the neuronal mechanisms that regulate eating behaviour). Pica is also related to early weaning in kittens, typically orphans, that have been raised by their owners and which often start the sucking behaviour when with their owners and then go on to chewing and ingesting different fabrics. Evidently, this behaviour is associated with a high level of patient anxiety.

DIAGNOSIS

The diagnosis is made using information provided by the owner during the anamnesis and by observing the patient's behaviour.

A differential diagnosis is necessary to distinguish pica from compulsive syndromes or cat stereotypies.

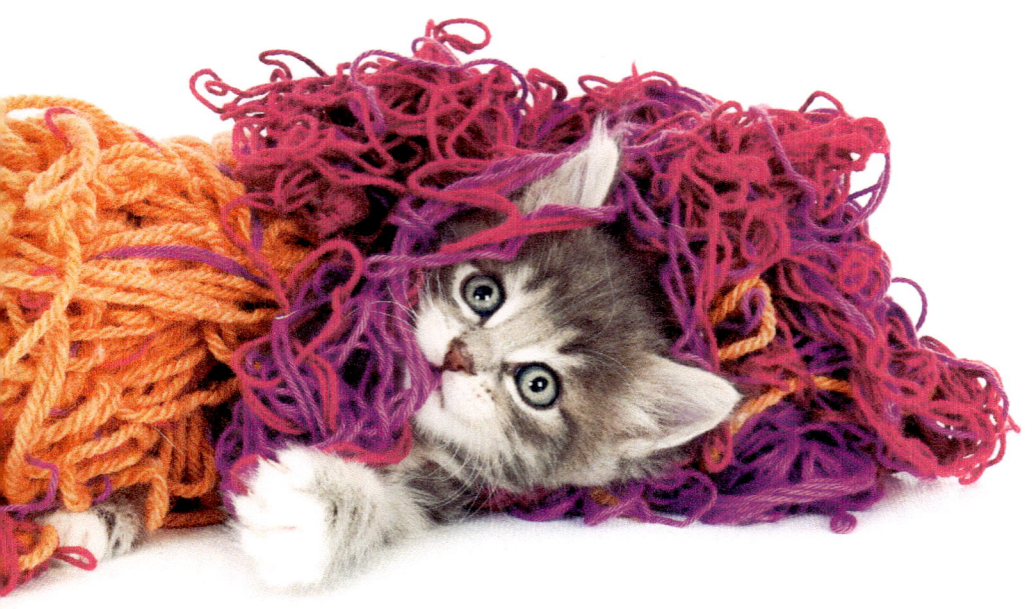

PROGNOSIS

The prognosis is guarded because cats are very strongly motivated to act out this behaviour and it is very hard to train them to stop despite the application of therapeutic measures. Generally, the best advice for owners is to be extremely careful not to leave clothes within the cat's reach whenever it is left unsupervised.

TREATMENT

➤ **Behavioural therapy:** consists of remote punishment when the cat exhibits the pica behaviour, but this is very difficult, as cats quickly learn not to suck or eat fabrics or objects in the presence of people and only do it when alone. Vets should also tell owners to discourage sucking behaviours when their cat is with them (many owners are endeared by this sucking habit when their pet is relaxed and purring on their lap, so they allow it to continue).

➤ **Drug treatment:** is limited to the use of the same medicines employed to treat stereotyped behaviours in cats:

  ➤ Buspirone*: 1–5 mg/cat/day, administered orally in two daily doses.
  ➤ Fluoxetine*: 0.5–1.0 mg/kg, every 24 h, orally.
  ➤ Amitriptyline: 2.5–5.0 mg/cat, every 12 h, orally.
  ➤ Clomipramine: 0.5–1.5 mg/cat, every 24 h, orally.
  ➤ Clonazepam*: 0.25–1.10 mg/cat, every 12 h, orally.

* The author's drugs of choice.

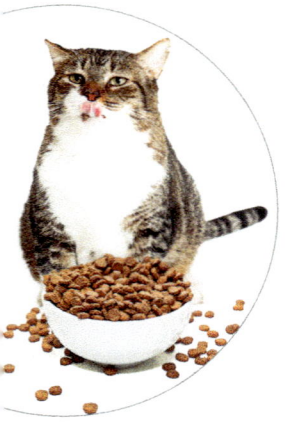

OBESITY

Obesity is the most common nutritional disorder observed in developed countries. While this statistic corresponds to humans, it can be translated to their pets. We now recognise obesity to be a behavioural disorder just like, for example, anorexia. Elderly animals and females are more susceptible to obesity, and castrated animals are probably more likely to suffer from it than intact individuals. Some studies in dogs have reported that certain breeds have a predisposition to obesity, but having said this, obesity is much less frequent in cats compared to dogs. It is hard to come across an obese cat, yet such cases do exist (Fig. 3).

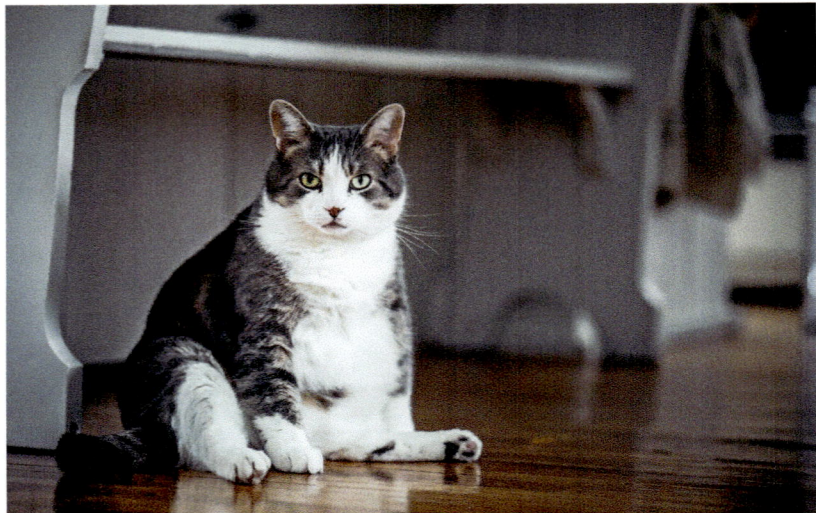

Figure 3. Obese cats are uncommon, but there are some examples.

DIAGNOSIS

A cat is considered obese when it exceeds its ideal body weight by 20 % (Fig. 4).

When trying to diagnose this behavioural disorder, identifying the cause of the obesity is much more important than determining whether or not the patient is obese. In most cases, the reason for the cat's obesity is related to how the owner feeds it, wherein incorrect practices generate poor eating habits.

PROGNOSIS

In general, and above all when the obesity results from poor eating habits due to the owner's feeding methods, the prognosis is highly favourable, so long as the owner is willing to amend their cat's dietary regimen.

TREATMENT

Obesity can be treated effectively if the owner is prepared to apply a strict, efficient, and intelligent approach to its treatment. It is essential that they change their pet's eating habits, and this applies to both the quantity and quality of the food the cat eats. Veterinary professionals should indicate low-calorie foods allotted in small amounts several times a day. This is very important, because unlike in the case of dogs, it is impossible to increase the patient's energy expenditure by increasing their level of daily exercise (e.g. by going for walks).

> Cats should never, under any circumstances, be indicated a fasting treatment because it could provoke severe liver disease.

Drug treatment, if necessary, is based on anxiolytic agents:
➤ Buspirone: 1–5 mg/cat/day, administered orally in two daily doses.
➤ Fluoxetine: 0.5–1.0 mg/kg, every 24 h, orally.

Figure 4	BODY CONDITION SCORE FOR CATS.

Too thin

1 Ribs visible in short-haired cats; no palpable fat; severe abdominal tuck; lumbar vertebrae and wings of ilia easily palpated.

2 Intermediate characteristics lying between body conditions 1 and 3.

3 Ribs easily palpable with minimal fat covering; lumbar vertebrae visible; waist is clearly visible behind ribs; minimal abdominal fat.

4 Intermediate characteristics lying between body conditions 3 and 5.

IDEAL

5 Well-proportioned; intercostal spaces visible; ribs palpable with slight fat covering; minimal abdominal fat.

Obese

6 Intermediate characteristics lying between body conditions 5 and 7.

7 Ribs not easily palpated with moderate fat covering; waist only just discernible; obvious rounding of abdomen; moderate deposit of abdominal fat.

8 Intermediate characteristics lying between body conditions 7 and 9.

9 Ribs not palpable under thick fat covering; abundant fat deposits over lumbar region, face, and limbs; abdominal distention with no waist; pronounced abdominal fat deposits.

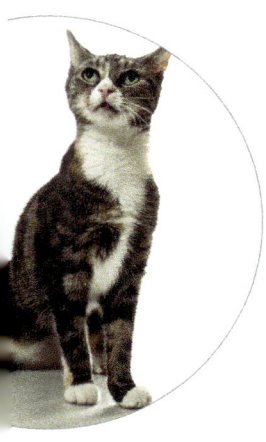

ANOREXIA

> Anorexia is the most commonly reported feeding disorder among domestic cats.

There are several possible causes of anorexia, which means it is hard to diagnose.

DIAGNOSIS

In cats, anorexia can be secondary to organic wasting diseases (feline retroviruses, neoplasms, etc.), a state of chronic stress due to an impoverished environment, or a smell disorder (the most typical are upper respiratory tract lesions due to viral infections).

It is important to remember that, as stated previously, cholecystokinin is actively involved in the neurological mechanisms that regulate eating behaviour.

Anorexia can be diagnosed through direct observation of the patient, complementary methods (blood tests, etc.), and by assessing the information collected during the anamnesis. Any patients that have not eaten for over 3 days can be considered as suffering anorexia and the absence of any clinical signs that would justify its appearance is indicative of a behavioural origin.

PROGNOSIS

The prognosis ranges from good to guarded, depending on the primary cause of the anorexia and whether or not it can be eliminated.

TREATMENT

The treatment of anorexia in cats should focus on addressing the underlying cause (whether environmental or organic). Behavioural therapy for anorexia consists of recommending environmental enrichment and reducing the patient's stress.

With respect to drug therapy, benzodiazepine anxiolytics can help treat anorexia (but must always be used with caution in cats, as mentioned already) because, besides mitigating the animal's anxiety and stress, they have appetite-stimulating properties (they are orexigenic). Another appetite-stimulating agent is cyproheptadine. Buspirone and fluoxetine can also be used to treat this behavioural problem.

➤ Diazepam: 0.2–0.5 mg/kg, every 12 or 24 hours, orally.
➤ Buspirone: 1–5 mg/cat/day, administered orally in two daily doses.
➤ Fluoxetine: 0.5–1.0 mg/kg, every 24 h, orally.
➤ Cyproheptadine: 1–2 mg/cat, every 12 h, orally.

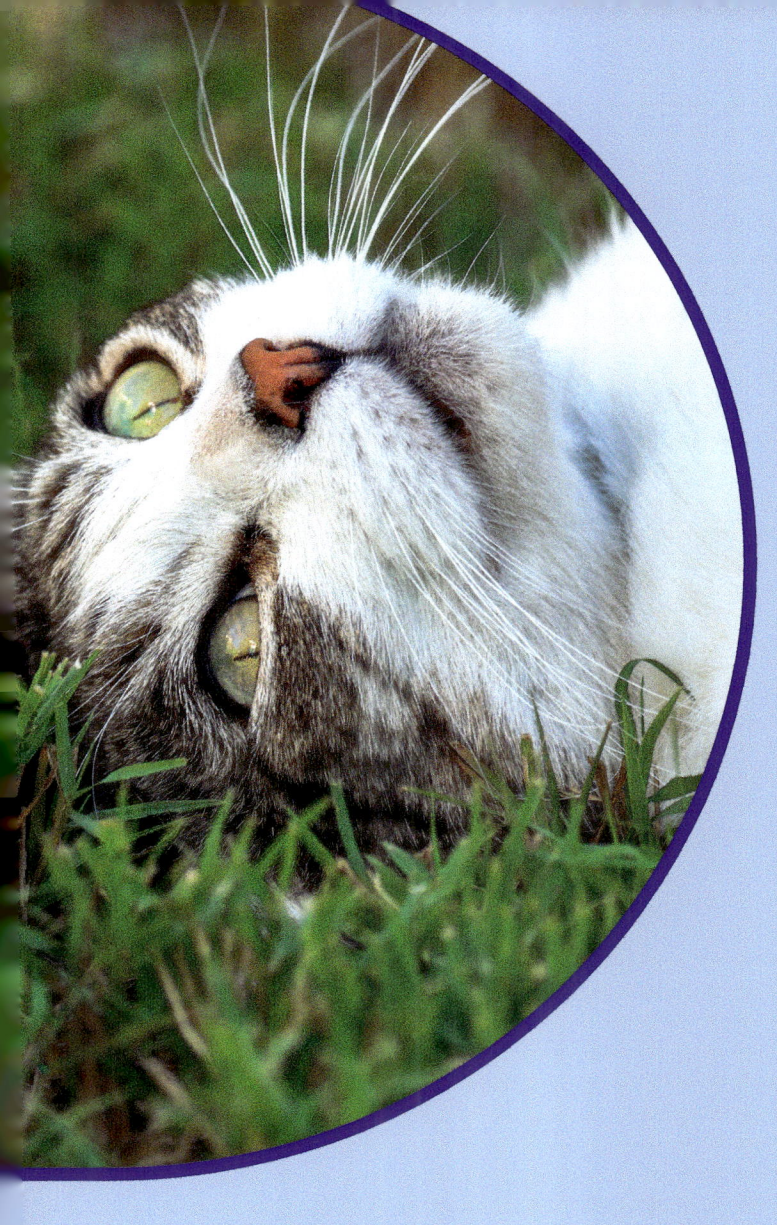

LATEST TREATMENT ADVANCES AND INNOVATIONS

INTRODUCTION

Without a shadow of a doubt, we are currently experiencing significant and rapid changes in many different disciplines. Veterinary medicine forms part of this panorama and therefore it also includes the study of animal behaviour or ethology.

The present chapter discusses recent advances made in the pharmacological treatment of behavioural disorders in cats.

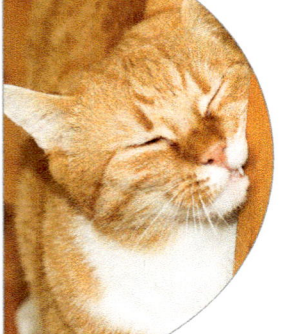

CAT PHEROMONES

Cat pheromones, which have been available and in use for several years now, have only recently experienced a surge in popularity and application to the treatment of behavioural disorders in house cats. To determine whether they are necessary in the treatment of cats with behavioural problems, first we must develop a clear understanding of their mechanism of action.

Pheromones are chemicals secreted by many different living beings and they produce predictable effects on the behaviour of the individual that receives them, as long as both animals belong to the same species.

They mainly have an impact on sexual, social, and territorial behaviour. The main natural sources of feline pheromones are vaginal exudates, urine, and secretions from skin glands, both sebaceous and apocrine sweat glands, located in the:
➤ Head: in the chin, around the mouth, and in the ear canals.
➤ Perineal area.
➤ Interdigital spaces.

This is why cats brush these body areas against objects and individuals with whom they have a positive social link. Cats mark these objects or individuals as a reminder that they are sources which generate a sense of wellbeing and security for the cat.

THE OLFACTORY SYSTEM OF CATS

Cats have anatomically and physiologically evolved over thousands of years. Their evolution has doted them with an extraordinary sense of smell, which is partly because they have developed a huge number of olfactory cells.

> Pheromones are very closely related to the olfactory system and they play an important role in cat behaviour.

To understand the mechanism of action of cat pheromones, we need to look at the anatomical region that houses the olfactory centre in a cat's brain (Fig. 1), as well as the location and function of the vomeronasal organ (or Jacobson's organ) (Fig. 2).

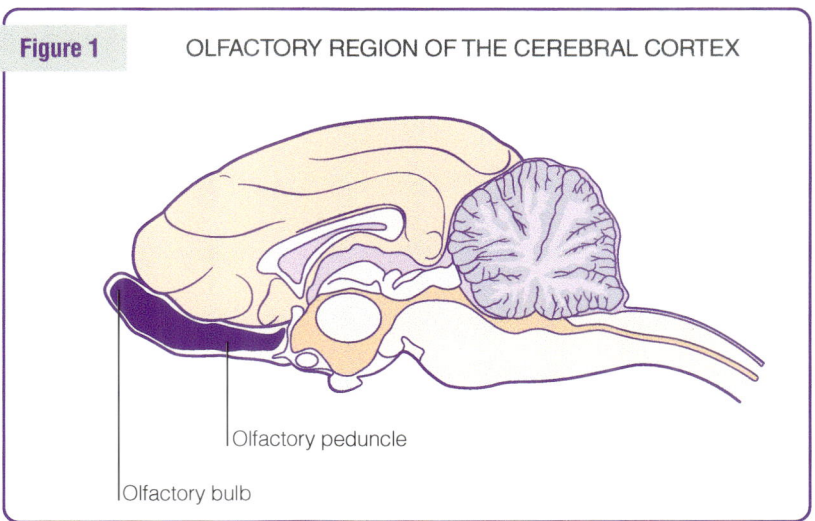

Figure 1   OLFACTORY REGION OF THE CEREBRAL CORTEX

Olfactory peduncle

Olfactory bulb

Medial view of the right cerebral hemisphere in cats.

BEHAVIOURAL DISORDERS IN CATS

A cat's olfactory system (Fig. 2) is perfectly adapted to its environment and is one of the main weapons in their arsenal as impeccable hunters. The inside of a cat's nose is populated with very thin bone lamellae that are covered by the olfactory epithelium – the epithelium is made up of millions of olfactory cells. The main function of the bone lamellae is to create a very large surface area to support even more olfactory mucosa, thus increasing the number of olfactory cells. Furthermore, the lamellae also ensure that air enters more slowly, transforming laminar flow into turbulent flow, hence any odouriferous molecules in the air are in contact with the cat's olfactory cells for longer. Contact with these molecules stimulates the olfactory cells, which then send the relevant information to the brain. This is because the olfactory epithelium, at the entrance to the nose, is interwoven with the olfactory nerve that conducts the information to the olfactory centre located in the cat's frontal lobe. Once the information reaches the olfactory centre, the neuronal interaction between the different areas of the brain mean the animal associates the odour with previous experiences, it may decide what they relate to, and finally select the appropriate behaviour in response. For example, if a cat recognises the odour as that of a female in heat, it will react with a different behaviour than if the discernible smell was associated with a type of prey.

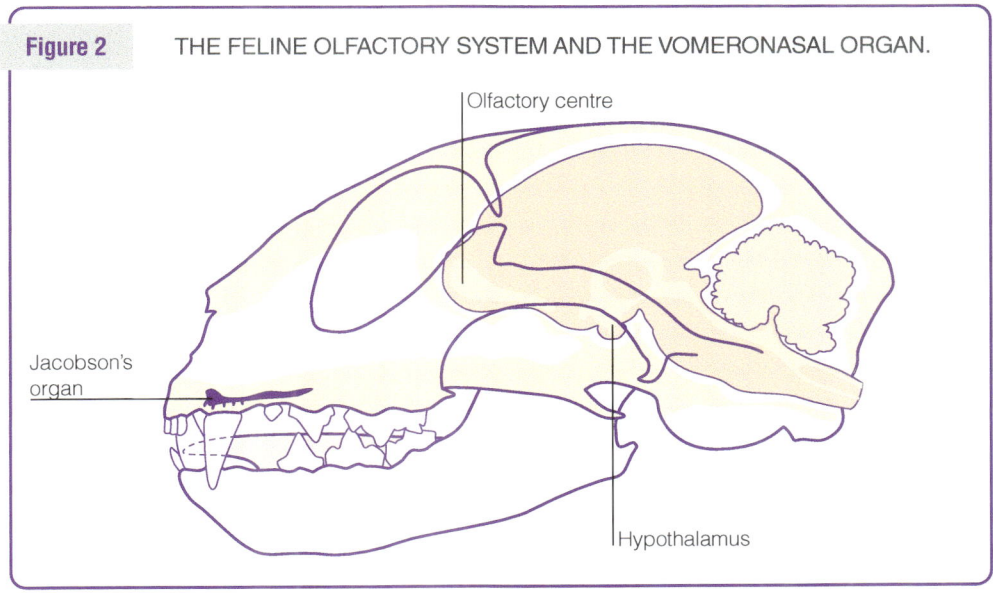

Figure 2   THE FELINE OLFACTORY SYSTEM AND THE VOMERONASAL ORGAN.

Olfactory centre

Jacobson's organ

Hypothalamus

In practice, cats perform what is called the flehmen response (Fig. 3), which is when a cat seems to bite the air, or open its mouth as if it were breathing through it. The flehmen response is normally associated with sniffing pheromones released by other cats. Cats do this so that the odouriferous particles come into contact with the vomeronasal organ and the nerve endings transmit the information to the brain's olfactory centre.

These anatomical and physiological references can help us better understand the function and utility of pheromones as therapeutic aids in the treatment of behavioural disorders in cats.

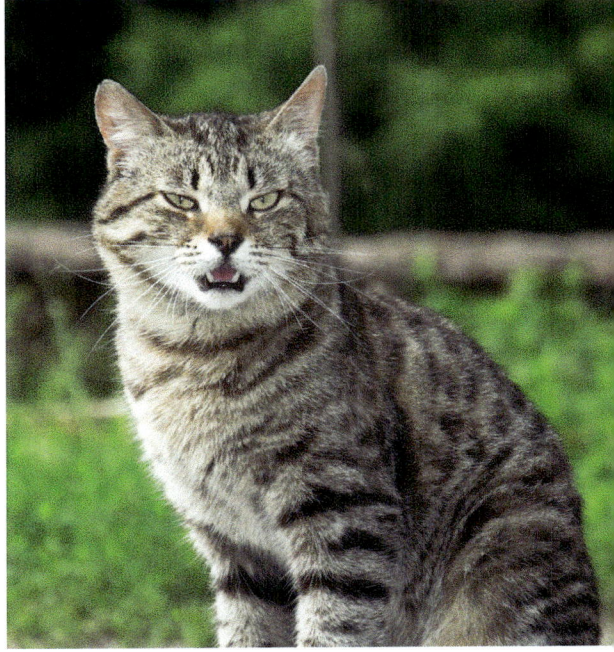

Figure 3. A cat displaying the flehmen response.

PHEROMONE CLASSIFICATION

According to their **mode of action** and effects, cat pheromones are classified as:

➤ Primer pheromones: produce slow and enduring changes in the recipient's reproductive physiology.

➤ Releaser pheromones: produce immediate but short-lived changes in the recipient. This is the type that generates feelings of wellbeing and calm in the recipient.

Based on their **chemical composition**, cat pheromones can be classified as:

➤ Volatile pheromones: are captured in the olfactory mucosa and are also releaser pheromones.

➤ Nonvolatile pheromones: are captured by the vomeronasal organ and fall into the primer category.

Feline pheromones have been associated with different parts of the body depending on the glands that secrete them and with the different situations in which cats release them. As such, from a behavioural point of view, the pheromones can be classified according to their **function**:

➤ Social pheromones: are used to identify other individuals within a social group. Cats secrete them by rubbing their cheeks, neck, or back against their owner's leg, another cat, or against an object. Accordingly, cats use a familiarisation pheromone to mark individuals or objects belonging to their familiar environment and which they associate with a state of wellbeing, calm, and security.

➤ Sex pheromones: are excreted along with sexual secretions and urine in order to establish contact with a member of the opposite sex and allow them to approach for mating purposes.

➤ Territorial pheromones: are released through urine and from interdigital glands in the paws. Evidently, they are used to mark territory.

➤ Alarm pheromones: are secreted from anal glands or sweat glands in the paw pads. Cats release them in tense situations, and they indicate that the cat is stressed or frightened.

➤ Appeasing pheromones: are released by female cats when nursing their kittens and help make the litter feel calm and secure.

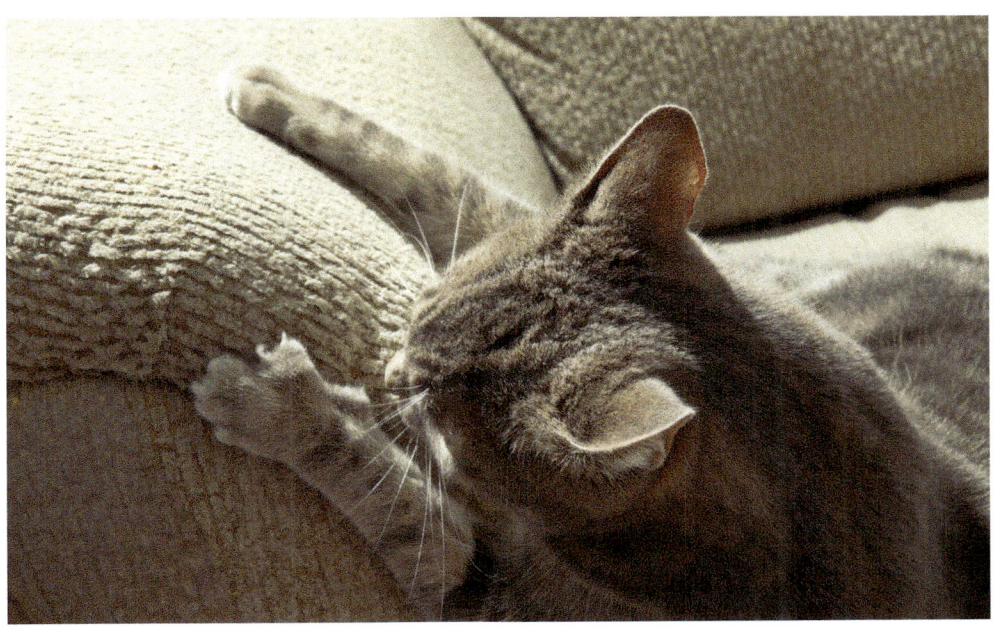

PHEROMONES IN THE TREATMENT OF BEHAVIOURAL DISORDERS IN CATS

The most used pheromones in veterinary medicine are synthetic analogues of social pheromones. They are recommended for a range of behavioural problems, but are most commonly prescribed to treat cases of territorial marking (using urine, faecal material, by scratching furniture, etc.). Pheromones are also indicated in certain situations of stress, for example, when handling a cat, during transport, when moving to a new house, and so on.

Cat pheromones are currently available in two formats: as room diffusers or sprays.

Room diffusers work well in cases where the balanced cohabitation between cats sharing the same house is upset for whatever reason or after moving to a new house, provided that the owner places a diffuser in the old house one month before moving and another in the new home.

> Synthetic pheromones are an excellent complement to most of the treatments indicated for the behavioural problems exhibited by pet cats.

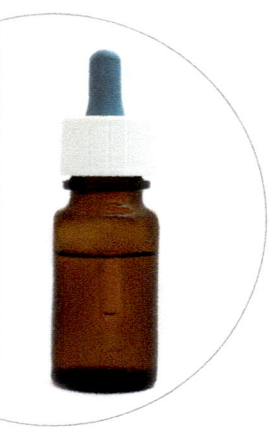

OTHER TREATMENT OPTIONS

Due to the increasing popularity of animal behaviour in the context of veterinary medicine, some new therapeutic options have been marketed recently that are essentially based on natural products. While all medicines, including psychoactive agents, are to some extent derivatives of natural products, society currently tends to prefer the use of products that are not recognised as psychoactive medicines. Therefore, the veterinary sector has started to produce medications in line with this tendency.

NATURAL MEDICINES

These are a group of medications that incorporate ingredients found in nature. They are based on a blend of plant extracts combined with different vitamins and amino acids such as L-tryptophan, which is an essential amino acid in the synthesis of serotonin that can only be obtained from food.

Given the importance of serotonin, it is only logical that any new products contain some essential amino acids, neurotransmitters (such as gamma-aminobutyric acid, or GABA), antioxidants, and plant extracts, which have all historically helped individuals relax.

> These products are available as drops or tablets for oral administration and are mainly indicated for stressful situations.

More complex medicines are available to treat elderly animals with cognitive dysfunction; besides antioxidants, vitamins, minerals, amino acids, and mitochondrial cofactors, they also incorporate coenzymes such as coenzyme Q10. There have been several studies into the role of nutrition in delaying the effects of ageing and the appearance of cognitive dysfunction. Acetylcholine is an important neurotransmitter involved in cognitive functions such as thought, learning, and memory. The ageing process causes a reduction in acetylcholine levels, while cell membranes lose fluidity and suffer damage due to free radicals and oxidation. Supplements such as antioxidants (vitamin E, vitamin C, selenium, etc.), polyunsaturated fatty acids, B-complex vitamins, and plant extracts improve the cognitive ability of any patients affected by ageing.

Some of the natural compounds with the greatest influence on the behaviour of household cats, which are often found in the ingredients of natural medicines used to support the treatment of behavioural disorders, include:

TRYPTOPHAN

The amino acid L-tryptophan is the metabolic precursor of serotonin, a neurotransmitter that plays an essential role in the regulation of mood, anxiety, appetite, and sleep. Once the body has absorbed L-tryptophan from the diet, it is converted into L-5-hydroxytryptophan by tryptophan hydroxylase (the rate-limiting enzyme in serotonin biosynthesis), which is then metabolised into 5-hydroxytryptamine or serotonin by decarboxylase.

Tryptophan must cross the blood–brain barrier before it can exert its effect; however, it has to compete with long-chain neutral amino acids (tyrosine, phenylalanine, valine, leucine, and isoleucine) that use the same transporters.

In food-producing animals, a diet supplemented with an optimal ratio of tryptophan and long-chain neutral amino acids reduces any stress and anxiety that may arise from the production conditions. It is therefore reasonable to assume that the same thing applies to household pets and particularly cats, as they are much more likely to suffer from the negative consequences of being confined (e.g. in indoor cats) considering their specific behavioural patterns (Fig. 4).

> Tryptophan-rich diets can induce a calming effect in cases of aggressiveness and tryptophan supplements can increase the feeling of wellbeing in some patients.

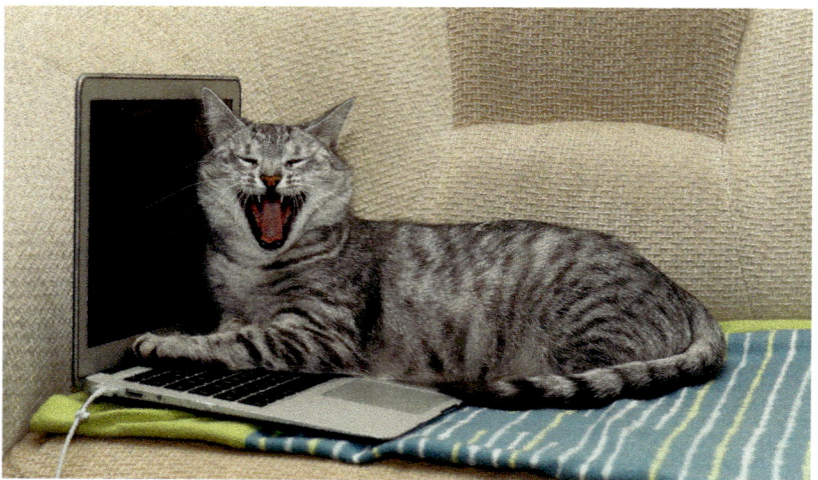

Figure 4. Some indoor cats may suffer stress and anxiety due to living in conditions of confinement. Tryptophan supplements can help minimise these clinical signs.

VITAMIN B$_3$

Vitamin B$_3$ is water soluble and easily incorporated into the diet. It affects metabolism by acting as the prosthetic group in coenzymes or a coenzyme precursor. Vitamin B$_3$ takes on two main forms, niacin (or nicotinic acid) and its amide form, nicotinamide.

Nicotinamide has a very similar physiological action on the central nervous system as the anxiolytic effects produced by benzodiazepines.

Its complementary use alongside the overall treatment forms a very helpful part of the therapeutic strategy implemented in patients with behavioural disorders.

THEANINE

L-Theanine is an amino acid found exclusively in green tea. While the molecule is not actually a sedative, it is responsible for the calming and relaxing effects associated with green tea. This is because it increases GABA levels (a neurotransmitter that is well-known for its ability to inhibit anxiety and stress-related disorders), reduces glutamate neurotoxicity, and has a positive effect on serotonin levels.

Cats tolerate L-theanine very well and it has known to have a calming effect.

There are other products based on a combination of L-theanine and L-tryptophan with plant extracts (such as *Piper methysticum* extracts) and B vitamins that act on the central nervous system. These products are available as tablets for oral administration.

α-CASOZEPINE

α-Casozepine is undoubtedly one of the most widely known nutraceutical substances.

α-Casozepine is a milk casein derivative (the α-S1-casein fraction), in this case, of bovine origin. It is available as tablets for oral administration, but it can also be incorporated as an ingredient in food (Fig. 5).

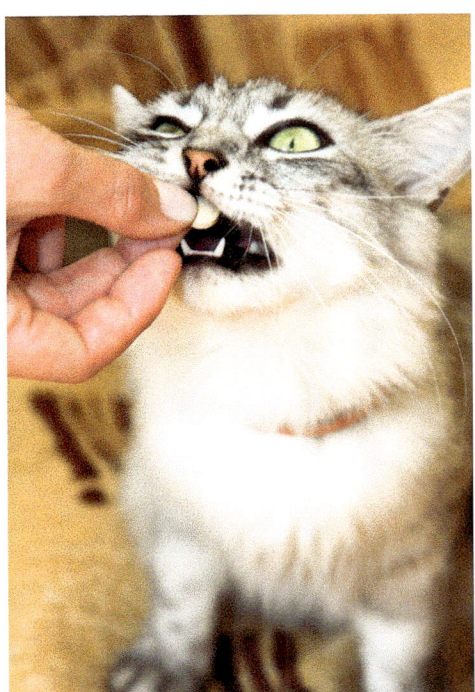

In nursing kittens, trypsin is the enzyme responsible for hydrolysing the casein in their mother's milk into α-casozepine, which binds with GABA receptors in the brain and produces a calming effect similar to that of diazepam, but without its side effects (sedation, lack of inhibition, and addiction). Cats have very good tolerance towards this natural relaxant, whether in its purest form, as a supplement, or a food ingredient.

As kittens grow their digestive system changes and tends to hydrolyse pepsin instead of casein, so adult cats only produce very small amounts of α-casozepine.

Figure 5. α-Casozepine can be administered as oral tablets or through the diet by using α-casozepine-supplemented foods.

> α-Casozepine has been used with good results to treat anxiety and stress-related symptoms.

α-Casozepine has a selective affinity for the benzodiazepine binding site in $GABA_A$ receptors in the brain, thus enhancing the effects of GABA.

When α-casozepine attaches to its specific binding site on the GABA receptor, it can increase GABA's affinity for its own neurorecepter. This increases the opening frequency of the associated chloride ion channels, resulting in GABA-induced hyperpolarisation of the axonal membrane and subsequently a reduction in the brain's postsynaptic neuronal activity. This enhances the inhibitory action of any available GABA and produces an anxiolytic effect.

α-Casozepine is useful at preventing anxiety in predictably stressful situations such as moving home, the arrival of a baby, changes in the owners' timetables, visits to the vet, and so on.

> α-Casozepine can be administered without any safety concerns, as it does not have any side effects or contraindications.

NUTRACEUTICALS

Nutraceuticals are functional foods that help improve a patient's quality of life, maintain them in good health, and prevent diseases. Therefore, foods enriched with vitamins and minerals, or which contain modified ingredients (fatty acids, fibre, etc.), can be considered nutraceutical products.

We now know that an individual's emotions, cognition, perception, mood, and so on, all depend on a very delicate balance between neurotransmitters and their receptors. Given that, through dietary intake, appropriate nutrition provides the right nutrients required to maintain a healthy nervous system in perfect working order, then it is reasonable to believe that diet also influences animal behaviour.

For this reason, the range of veterinary nutrition products now includes different types of functional foods indicated for specific behavioural alterations (aggressiveness, anxiety, stress). These products contain a correctly balanced blend of essential nutrients that represent important supplements in the treatment of behavioural problems.

THE IMPORTANCE OF ACTIVE OWNER PARTICIPATION

Complementary therapies must be used to supplement the conventional treatment of behavioural disorders in pet cats.

This is an important point that owners must take on board, not only with respect to products of natural origin used in complementary therapies, but also regarding the use of allopathic psychoactive drugs. Otherwise, owners might not be inclined to participate or get actively involved in their pet's behavioural therapy, which is an extremely important factor when it comes to resolving behavioural disorders, as it is the owner who must implement the environmental changes and behaviour modification techniques indicated by the veterinary surgeon.

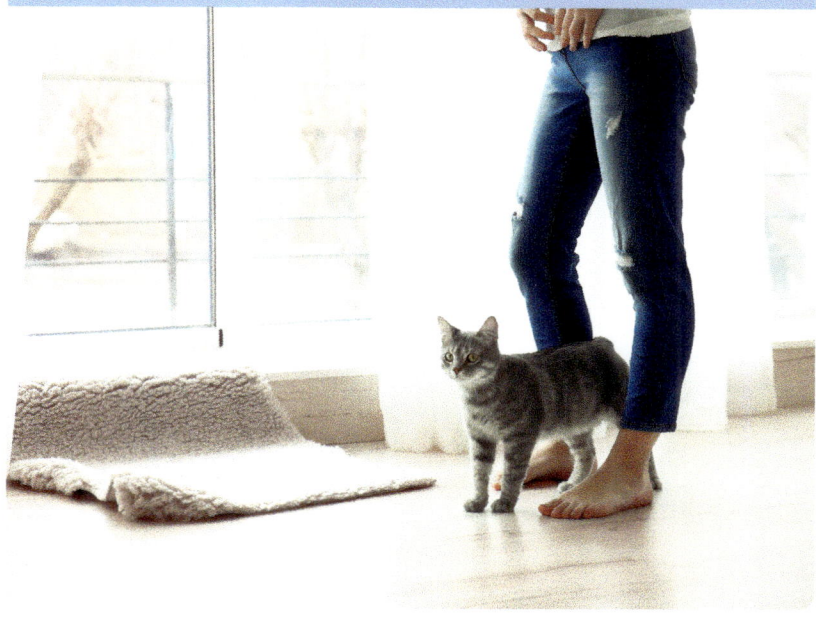

BIBLIOGRAPHY

BEATA C, BEAUMONT-GRAFF E, COLL V ET AL. Effect of alpha-casozepine (Zylkene) on anxiety cats, Journal of Veterinary Behaviour, 2007, 2, 40–46.

BEATA C, BEAUMONT-GRAFF E, DIAZ C ET AL. Effects of alpha-casozepine (Zylkene) versus selegiline hydrochloride (Selgian, Anipryl) on anxiety disorders in dogs, *Journal of Veterinary Behavior*, 2007, 2, 175-183.

BEAVER BV. *Canine Behavior: A guide for Veterinarians*, Saunders Company, Philadelphia, 1999.

BEAVER BV. *Feline Behavior: A guide for Veterinarians*, Saunders Company, Philadelphia, 1992.

BEAVER BV. *Veterinary Aspects of Feline Behavior*, The CV Mosby Company, St. Louis, 1980, 168–174.

BEAVER BV. Disorders of Behavior, in *The Cat: Diseases and Clinical Management* , SHERDING, R ET AL., Churchill Livingston, New York, 1989, 163–184.

BEEBE AD, OVERALL KL. Feline behavioral disorders, in *Handbook of Veterinary Internal Medicine,* MORGAN RV, Churchill Livingston, New York, 1997.

BERNSTEIN KS. A physiological reason for defecating outside the litterbox, *Vet Med Small Animal Clinic*, 1977; 72:1549.

BORCHELT PL. Cat elimination behavior problems, *Veterinary Clinics of North America: Small Animal Practice*, 1991, 21, 257–264.

BRUNO R. Geriatría conductual, chapter 83, in *Consulta rápida en la clínica diaria*, MUCHA CJ, SORRIBAS CE, PELLEGRINO FC, Intermédica, Buenos Aires, 2005.

BRUNO R. Comportamientos estereotipados, in *Medicina Felina Práctica II*, MINOVICH FG, PALUDI AE, AUTRAN DE MORAIS H, Royal Canin Argentina, 2004.

CHANDLER EA. *Medicina y terapéutica caninas*, Editorial Acribia, Zaragoza, 1986.

DODMAN N, SHUSTER L. *Psicofarmacología de los trastornos del comportamiento animal*, Intermédica, Buenos Aires, 2000.

HALIP J. *Feline elimination problems*, Presentation at AVMA, San Francisco, 994.

HART BL, HART LA, BAIN MJ. *Canine & Feline Behavioral Therapy*, Blackwell Publishing, Oxford, 2006.

HART BL, HART LA. *Canine and Feline Behavioral Therapy*, Lea & Febiger, Philadelphia, 1985, 134-136.

LANDSBERG G, HUNTHAUSEN W, ACKERMAN L. *Manual de problemas de conducta del perro y gato*, Editorial Acribia, Zaragoza, 1998.

LORENZ K. *Cuando el hombre encontró al perro*, Tusquets Editores SA, Barcelona, 1984.

MANTECA X. *Etología clínica veterinaria del perro y del gato*, Multimédica, Barcelona, 2003.

MORRIS D. *Guía para comprender a los perros*, Emecé Editores, Barcelona, 1988.

O´FARRELL V. *Manual of Canine Behaviour*, British Small Animal Veterinary Association, Gloucester, 1996.

OVERALL KL. *Clinical Behavioral Medicine for Small Animals*, The CV Mosby Company, St. Louis, 1997, 161-194.

PAGEAT P, BEATA C, *Curso de etología clínica,* Society of Veterinary Surgeons Specialists in Small Animals, Santiago de Chile, 2000.

PELAEZ DEL HIERRO F, VEA BARÓ J. *Etología, bases biológicas de la conducta animal y humana*, Ediciones Pirámide, Madrid, 1997.

VOITH V, BORCHELT P. *Readings in Companion Animal Behavior*, Veterinary learning systems, Trenton, 1996.

PHOTOGRAPHY CREDITS

Ricardo Luis Bruno Cazeaux: págs. 11 (superior), 26, 27, 30 (inferior), 32, 34 (superior), 37, 40, 52, 55, 58, 63, 70, 85 (inferior), 91, 92, 96, 114 (izquierda), 127, 134 (inferior), 137, 141, 143, 152, 153 (derecha), 157, 159, 163, 170, 180

SHUTTERSTOCK.COM

4 PM production: pág. 159

Africa Studio: págs. 45, 122, 144, 213

Alex Zotov: pág. 18 (superior)

Alexander Demyanov: pág. 134

Alona Cherniakhova: pág. 35 (superior)

Amelia Martin: pág. 94

Ammit Jack: pág. 41

ANATOLY Foto: pág. 24

anetapics: pág. 34 (inferior)

Anurak Pongpatimet: págs. 6, 154 (izquierda)

Benoit Daoust: pág. 196 (inferior)

bmf-foto.de: pág. 202

Boryana Manzurova: pág. 47

Catherine Murray: pág. 207

Cavan-Images: pág. 99

charnsitr: pág. 77 (superior)

Ching Louis Liu: pág. 77 (inferior)

Christin Lola: pág. 89

claire norman: pág. 90

Cristina Conti: pág. 104

cunaplus: pág. 51

cynoclub: págs. 133, 174

D.Bond: pág. 185

Dan Breckwoldt: pág. 14

De Jongh Photography: pág. 194

DibaniMedia: pág. 199

Dietmar Oelke: pág. 135

Doucefleur: pág. 156

Ege Tascioglu: pág. 35 (inferior)

Elenica: pág. 211

Eric Isselee: pág. 130

Ermolaev Alexander: pág. 140

FannyF: pág. 85 (superior)

German Nareklishvili: pág. 192

Guitarfoto studio: pág. 125

Imageman: pág. 208

iprachenko: pág. 110

JakubD: pág. 166

Jaromir Chalabala: pág. 57

Javier Brosch: pág. 43

Johann Knox: pág. 93

Joyce Vincent: pág. 154 (derecha)

Kapustin Igor: pág. 167

Karpova: pág. 186

Kenton D. Gomez: pág. 5

Kim Christensen: pág. 83

komkrit Preechachanwate: pág. 78

Kuttelvaserova Stuchelova: pág. 115

Lenti Hill: pág. 98

lightpoet: pág. 113

Luke23: pág. 4

Massimiliano Agati: pág. 36

Published by Grupo Asís Biomedia SL